Books by Mildred Tengbom

Is Your God Big Enough?

The Bonus Years

Table Prayers

Fill My Cup, Lord (with Dr. Luverne C. Tengbom)

A Life to Cherish

Especially for Mother

Bible Readings for Families (with Dr. Luverne C. Tengbom)

Sometimes I Hurt

Help for Bereaved Parents

Help for Families of the Terminally Ill

Does Anyone Care How I Feel?

I Wish I Felt Good All the Time

No Greater Love: The Story of Clara Maass

Why Waste Your Illness?

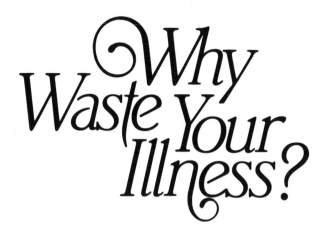

Why Waste Your Illness?

Let God
Use It for Growth.

Mildred
Tengbom

AUGSBURG Publishing House • Minneapolis

WHY WASTE YOUR ILLNESS?
Let God Use It for Growth

Library of Congress Cataloging in Publication Data

Tengbom, Mildred.
    WHY WASTE YOUR ILLNESS?

    1. Sick—Religious life.   2. Sick—Prayer-books and devotions—English.   I. Title.
BV4910.T46   1984   248.8'6   83-72113
ISBN 0-8066-2057-9 (pbk.)

Manufactured in the U.S.A.   APH 10-7182

   2   3   4   5   6   7   8   9   0   1   2   3   4   5   6   7   8   9

To my daughter Judy
and to my nieces: Susan, Mary Beth, Carolyn, and Ann,
committed to careers of health care,
one as a medical technologist,
two as doctors, one as a nurse, and one as a dental technician

Contents

My sincere thanks to all who answered questionnaires and who granted interviews. Special thanks go to four people who graciously and carefully critiqued my manuscript and offered helpful suggestions: Hazel M. Johnson, Ph.D., professor emeritus, Gustavus Adolphus College, formerly chairman, department of nursing; the Rev. Gregg Selander, chaplain, St. Mary's Hospital, Long Beach, Calif.; Jeanne Crumley, musician, who encountered and overcame a bout with cancer; and Eileen Guder Triplett, writer, author, and friend.

Preface

Generally speaking I think of myself as a healthy person with an abundance of energy. Consequently when my editor asked me to consider writing a book on illness, I hesitated. Should I be the one to address this topic?

However, I was surprised, as I reflected, to count 19 times that I had entered the hospital. On some of these occasions I had undergone major surgery. In addition, during my years in India and Africa I had suffered from malaria, dysenteries, and dengue fever. In the United States I had mumps as an adult, as well as pneumonia, and once I was involved in an automobile accident. I realized that in spite of being a healthy person I have had numerous encounters with illness.

Yet I still hesitated. Although I have experienced three fairly close brushes with death, none of my illnesses has been protracted, of a life-threatening or crippling nature, or has involved unrelieved, continuous, severe pain. I have friends who suffer and have suffered in these ways, and often I have stood silent by their sides, not knowing what to say.

What then would I have to say in a book on the subject of illness?

However, a number of my suffering friends have shown me how it is possible, with God's help, to triumph in illness. They believe that we should not waste our illnesses. What is gained, they ask, by complaining, chafing, resisting, grumbling, or becoming bitter? Although illness deprives us of some control, we still retain the power to determine what our illness will do to us as persons. My friends say they have come to appreciate their illnesses. Time in bed, in the hospital, and at home, and the care of medical attendants and family have helped them discover new values, develop a deeper faith in God, and grow in love and compassion. So rather than waste your illness, they suggest that you accept it as a gift—an opportunity that God can use for your growth.

This book invites you to let God do just that.

Illness
Thank God for quietude—
A time to rest from frenzied haste,
For making clear evaluations and comparisons.

Thoughts stored up and pushed aside
In the busy whirl of life
Now rush and tumble before me,
Begging to be noticed,
Like children—eager, asking for attention.

And so I let them pass by in review—
Weighing, sifting, choosing.
Those I thought I must hold fast
I find myself discarding;
And thoughts that I had put away
To be forgotten,
I ask them now to live again.
GERTRUDE HANSON

I'm Sick!

"The best laid schemes o' mice and men
Gang aft a-gley."

How often my husband has quoted these words of Robert
Burns to me. And now it's happened again. I'm sick, and all
my plans are interrupted.

I hadn't planned on getting sick. I most surely do not like
it. But it has occurred to me that maybe this time I shouldn't
waste my illness. Wouldn't it be better if I asked God what
he has for me to learn during this time?

But in order to learn I'll have to start out with the right
attitude. Some attitudes won't help.

For example, sometimes I've taken illness in a matter-of-
fact way: "Everybody gets ill from time to time. No big deal.
It will pass."

Yes, most of the time it passes, and health returns. But
with that attitude I've gained little else besides restored
health.

17

I've tried the role of the stoic too: "Don't tell anybody I'm going to have surgery." "I don't need medication (even if I am hurting)." That attitude not only does not yield me anything, it depletes me. I cut myself off from the love and support friends would give me, and I suffer unnecessarily.

I've also tried my hand at being a martyr: "I'll carry on with the housework if it kills me." The effects of such an attitude both on me and others are so miserable I don't even want to think about them.

I've been manipulative too. After all, taking care of four kids and entertaining guests can make one very tired. Lying in bed, even if one is ill, can be simply delicious, and the temptation to extend the illness to get a little more attention is enticing.

Playing sick when quibbling among the children gets more than one feels one can bear is tempting too. I remember one harassed mother of four who escaped so completely she had to have psychiatric help to bring her back.

I had an elderly friend who tried to alleviate her loneliness by alarming me with gasping phone calls, claiming she was having a heart attack. But when I arrived at her home, almost always I found her composed and able to walk around, only wanting company. It got to the point that I never knew whether the "attack" was real or simulated.

Our personalities are so complex and our hearts so in love with ourselves that we can enjoy being sick because of the benefits we gain. That's being manipulative with illness. The trouble is, sooner or later, people will discover what we are doing and abandon us. Later, if we really become ill, they might not believe us. Playing "wolf, wolf" by pretending to be ill when we are not or pretending to be more ill than we are grants us only temporary gratification, and later we lose more than we gain.

Nursing resentment, anger, or self-pity doesn't help either. Goodness knows, I've done that: "Why do I have to be sick again?" "Why does it have to be *me?*" "Now my plans are all messed up! It isn't fair!" Being resentful or pouring self-pity over ourselves not only doesn't help; it actually hinders. It prevents healing. When we are resentful or angry, our body responds in ways not conducive to healing. We're not happy; our bodies aren't happy. And when we're feeling this way, we usually see to it that nobody around us is happy either.

Apathy won't help us either, docile and harmless as it may seem to be. Apathy actually holds the power of ending life for us. Deeply depressed after the death of our second little son who had been born prematurely, I slipped into apathy. My body responded with a high temperature that could not be traced to any physical cause. Only when my doctor talked to me in such a way that I became angry and began to talk back did the temperature disappear. Later he apologized, but then explained, "I had to do something to get you to begin to fight."

Some of my acquaintances insist illness is an attack of the Evil One. Once when a muscle spasm pulled together two deteriorated discs in my neckbone, pinching a nerve in between, I had to resort to wearing a neck collar. A woman who saw me whispered in my ear, "I know what you're up against. It's an attack of the devil. Resist him. Throw him out, and your neck will be all right." Maybe. It's possible, I guess, that the Evil One can attack us physically, and suffering on a massive scale seems to be occasioned by an evil force. But when illness disables me, I'd rather look for the Lord in that circumstance than Satan.

So then, rather than persisting in any of these attitudes, how much better if I engage my illness in battle and marshal all the forces I can to recover. At the same time I will seek to be teachable. I shall actively try to be alert to hear God's voice and learn all I can from God and from others. And I will stubbornly maintain an attitude of faith, believing that God can do something in me and through me during this experience.

Helps for Your Quiet Times with the Lord

We acquaint ourselves with what the Lord says

Read Isaiah 40:27-31. What does the writer declare we often say when things go wrong for us? What does the writer assure us God is like? What promises are there for us in these verses?

Read Isaiah 45:9. What characterizes a proper relationship to God?

Read Isaiah 63:9-10. Note the verbs in 63:9. What has God done? What is the significant first word in verse 10? To what does the writer equate rebelling against God?

Read 1 John 1:9.

We reflect and meditate

I haven't the right to choose the wood of my cross.

MICHEL QUOIST

When Thou callest me to go through the dark valley, let me not persuade myself that I know a way around.　　JOHN BAILLE

What is the greatest evil of suffering? Not the suffering itself but our rebellion against it, the state of interior revolt which often accompanies it.　　JEAN GROU

20

We pray

O Divine Spirit,
who in all the events of life art knocking at the door of my heart,
help me to respond to Thee.
I would take the events of my life as good and perfect gifts from
　　Thee.
I would receive even the sorrows of life as disguised gifts from
　　Thee.
I would have my heart open at all times to receive;
　　　at morning, noon, and night,
　　　in spring and summer and winter.
Whether Thou comest to me in sunshine or in rain
　　　I would take Thee into my heart joyfully.
Thou art Thyself more than sunshine;
Thou art Thyself compensation for the rain.
It is Thee, and not Thy gifts I crave.
Knock, and I shall open to Thee.　GEORGE MACDONALD

The Stranger
I Live With

Augustine once commented: "Men go abroad to wonder at the height of mountains, at the huge waves of the sea, at the long courses of the rivers, at the vast compass of the ocean, at the circular motion of the stars; and they pass by themselves without wondering."

Illness can afford us the opportunity to learn more about our bodies, and, as we do, to develop a deeper sense of awe. We also can use this time to learn how to use better the faculties God has given us.

Following a trip to Asia I was plagued with what the hill people of the Himalayas call "internal landslides." Attacks became more frequent and violent, finally driving me to a doctor. By then I was so weak and dizzy that I couldn't even sit up. An hour later, as I lay in a hospital bed, a medical attendant wheeled in an apparatus to monitor my heart. I protested it wasn't my heart that was causing problems; it was my digestive system. The attendant smiled benevolently and tolerantly and quietly went on with his tests.

Later as I lay watching the intravenous fluid drip into my veins, my doctor came in. I was seriously dehydrated, he said. I had stopped eating and drinking, thinking this would stop my diarrhea, but it instead had caused severe dehydration. Dehydration, he explained, allows the red corpuscles to remain in the blood, but the vessels constrict. The heart labors to pump the thickened blood. Deaths that occur during heat waves, he explained, frequently are the results of heart attacks that have been caused by dehydration. The reason they had monitored my heart was because they wanted to know how it had responded to the strain.

The body, he went on, tries to relieve the heart by extracting the fluid from the tissues so the blood can flow more freely but in doing so drains away the potassium, leaving one without energy. He motioned to the intravenous apparatus. Potassium was now flowing into my system along with the fluid to replace what had been lost.

As I listened to my doctor, I marveled at the domino effect illness has on the body. When one part ceases to function properly, often another part breaks down, and soon it seems everything has gone wrong.

Another time I was apprehensive that a retina in my right eye was becoming detached. As my doctor kept watch over it, my curiositly led me to reading a little about our eyes.

We say, "I saw it with my own eyes." Do we? No. Rather our brain interprets what waves of light are imprinting on our eyes. For example, when vibrations of 450 million million a second hit the retinal surface, the color of red is conveyed to the brain. When the vibrations are 750 million million a second, the brain interprets the color as violet.

But how marvelous that my brain is able simultaneously to interpret accurately all that is being imprinted on the retina of my eye. Colors of every hue are kept sharply delineated from one another. Movement. Particles. Objects. Shapes. And expressions. Through the impressions on the retina the brain continuously interpets all.

How casual we are about our ability to see. Illness can afford us opportunities to sharpen our skills of seeing. How much do you see? Can you describe the hospital attendants who have come to your bedside? Would you be able to recognize them if you saw them again someplace else? What are the colors of the walls in your room? How long has it been since you really looked carefully into the faces and eyes of your loved ones? Have new wrinkles appeared? Are there lines of weariness? What do their eyes tell you? What about the visitors who come to you? What do you see in their faces?

As you lie in bed, learn to look. You can practice the art of observation also by opening a travel magazine or a book of paintings.

Marvelous as our vision is, we know we have limitations. There are things in space around us that our eyes are not seeing. Sometimes when I have thought about this, it has helped me grasp the fact that God is invisible and unseen. God has promised to be with us, but we do not see God. The disciples were fortunate in seeing Christ appear in visible form after the resurrection. And we have his promise that we too shall see him as he is. So is it possible that if our eyes weren't limited we could see him with us even now?

Even as our eyes are limited, so are our ears. Have you ever marveled at how our ears mercifully shut out most of the noise in the universe around us? They do not pick up all those myriad sounds that the telephone, radio, and TV can make audible to us at our will. We hear, and yet there are many things we do not hear.

How much do you hear? Use your time of recuperation to learn to listen. What sounds have you heard since you awakened this morning? What sounds do you hear now? Put on a record or tape of classical music. Listen. Try to identify the different musical instruments. Listen to the tones of those who talk to you. Try to describe the sounds you hear: "as harsh as _____," "as soft as _____."

Or take our sense of smell. Most of us smell very little. James Mitchell, who was born blind and deaf, could smell when a stranger came into the room. It is said that Peruvian Indians, in the darkness of the night, could tell what race of person was approaching them. Smell your hands. Smell the sheets of your bed, your toothpaste. Smell anything that is within range of your smelling powers. Recall smells. Develop this marvelous sense God has given you.

How conscious are you of touch? Paul Tournier laments that the cold, impersonal steel of instruments has replaced the warm touch of a physician's hand. Who of us who has been seriously ill cannot recall how much it has meant to have someone touch us?

Helen Keller developed her sense of touch to the point that she felt the impact the universe made on the cells of her skin. She could write of how welcome the "tactile silence" (the silence that could be felt) of the country was after the din of the town and "the irritating concussions of the train." She spoke of how "noiseless and undisturbing are the demolition, repairs and alterations of nature compared to those humans undertake."

We might not be able to develop our sense of touch as it concerns our entire body surface to that sensitive degree, but we surely can become more conscious of what touch means to us. How do you clasp the hand of another? What does your handclasp mean? How do you touch others? How do they touch you?

Helen Keller told of how her dog loved her as he touched

her. "He pressed close to me as if he were fain to crowd himself into my hand. He loved me with his tail, with his paw, with his tongue. If he could speak, I believe he would say with me that paradise is attained with touch; for in touch is all love and intelligence."

The Nepali people of the Himalayas have a quaint exchange of remarks when they meet each other out for a walk.

"Where are you going?" one asks.

"I'm out to eat some air," is the reply.

Accurate and perceptive. For while we can get along without food for many days and without water for less, we cannot get along without "eating air" for more than a few minutes. Our lives are intertwined inexorably, not only with other people, but with animals and with all nature.

Even though the psalmist's knowledge of the universe and the human body was much more limited than ours, still he was caught up in a sense of awe and wonder when he wrote Psalm 8. First he comments on the immensity and wonder of the universe. But then he asks, "What is man that you are mindful of him, the son of man that you care for him?" I can almost see him shaking his head as he continues, "You made him a little lower than the heavenly beings and crowned him with glory and honor."

Helps for Your Quiet Times with the Lord

We acquaint ourselves with what the Lord says

Read 1 Corinthians 6:19. Underline what you consider to be the key words in this verse. What does this verse tell us about the regard God has for our bodies? What does this verse tell us about how close God is to us?

Memory is an invaluable gift. But remembering can also bring regrets. What does God say he will not remember? (Isa. 43:25; Heb. 8:12.) What can we remember that will help us? (Ps. 63: 1-8; Lam. 3:19-26; 31-33.)

We reflect and meditate

With the wonderful eye of love God and man behold one another.   KAGAWA

God gave us memory that we might have roses in December.
JAMES M. BARRIE

One of the saddest experiences which can come to a human being is to awaken, gray-haired and wrinkled, near the close of an unproductive career, to the fact that all through the years he or she has been using only a small part of himself or herself.
V. W. BURROWS

We pray

Thank God for your marvelous body. Mention specific parts as you give thanks. Thank God for the gift of life.

Thank God for dwelling in you. Lie quietly and feel God's life permeating your whole being.

What's Happening to Me?

"You're behaving like a baby!"

The weary wife, who had been running up and down the stairs for weeks, caring for her recuperating husband, finally exploded.

She was right. Her husband had been behaving like a baby. When she brought him orange juice, he wanted water. When she brought him water, it wasn't cold enough. When she turned on the air conditioner, he complained that the room was too cold. When she turned it down, he grumbled that it was too hot. When she shooed the kids out of the house because he said they were too noisy, he said he couldn't stand the quietness. When his partner called to ask for advice, he asked why people couldn't let a sick man alone. But when he heard of decisions being made without consulting him, he fumed. No one could please him. He *was* acting like a spoiled kid.

It's not unusual. Illness affects, not only our bodies, but our personalities as well. One of the most common changes that takes place is that we revert to childish behavior and reactions. Almost all of us, for example, get scared.

A cartoon strip shows Dennis in bed between his mother and father, blanket pulled up to his chin. "A little thunder doesn't scare me," he says. "It's just a *lot* of thunder that makes me afraid."

So too with illness. Colds, sore throats, and flu we can tolerate. But when we become more seriously ill, we get afraid. Are men even more susceptible to this? Often they fuss and want to keep taking their temperatures. They are worried about their blood pressure. They're sure they are going to die. At the same time they stubbornly may refuse to take medication or follow the doctor's orders—acting again like children. Still not only men, but all of us suffer from feeling scared when we are sick. We need a lot of holding, loving, and encouraging. We need someone strong alongside us who will protect, reassure, and take care of us.

If our illness lands us in the hospital, our feelings of insecurity may be heightened simply because we lack one person with whom we can communicate on a regular basis. Perhaps our family physician has referred us to a specialist, who may call in other specialists. Nurses' schedules change so frequently we may not see the same nurse more than two or three times, and some nurses we may see only once. Also, with the varied uniforms worn, we may have difficulty identifying the nurses. This also produces a feeling of helplessness, frustration, and insecurity.

These feelings of insecurity can cause us to react in different ways. Sometimes we get crabby, or hard to please. We may complain about food or service, because at least this brings someone to our bedside, someone who will listen to us. A few explode in anger.

A few become meekly submissive, asking no questions,

making no requests and following all orders docilely. This can be dangerous, because even health professionals make mistakes.

Others refuse to part with the security of their known world. They arrive at the hospital with briefcase, tape recorder, clipboard and pen, set up office, and begin to use the phone.

Others try to compensate for feelings of insecurity by establishing close relationships with their doctor and nurses, closer even than with their family.

For some, nurses become mother figures, and this in itself encourages them to slip back into childish ways. For others even aged parents become, once again, significant supporters and morale boosters.

Becoming childlike again frees many of adult inhibitions. They then do things that may embarrass visitors or family and later cause them to blush when they recall what they said or did.

I remember a roommate whose baby had been stillborn. Before a room full of visitors she described in detail her labor and delivery. She went on to complain of the discomfort her swelling breasts were causing her and proceeded to display them.

And many Americans still can recall the picture of former President Lyndon Johnson pulling up his shirt to display the long incision on his paunchy abdomen.

Others react in the opposite way and become prudish to an extreme, even in front of their spouses.

Quite likely we also will find mixed feelings chasing around inside us. We're relieved to be in the hospital, but we also wish we were home. We enjoy being cared for, but we chafe under restricted freedom. "Why can't I do what I want?" we fume. "I hate being so helpless!" We are relieved of some pain, but then subjected to even more. We had hoped to rest, but discover how difficult it is to get unbroken sleep in a hospital.

Tempers and tears may overflow quickly. One woman, whose husband had been so self-controlled she had never realized he felt anger, was upset and distressed when she saw him lash out again and again in anger. Another woman was amazed at how jealous her husband became when she visited with and seemed to enjoy his roommate.

Family secrets also frequently are told to roommates. Husbands and wives are discussed. Trouble spots in marriages are shared, grievances aired.

A positive change that often takes place when people are ill is that sickness seems to soften many. Quite readily and genuinely they will say, "I'm sorry." They may be eager to provide for the comfort of others. A prayer or a Bible verse may trigger tears. A gift of flowers may produce profuse thanks. Cards are handled lovingly and read over and over. Parents will want to tell medical or housekeeping staff about their children and show pictures.

If, however, pain is troublesome, or if excessive tests have yielded no clues and the patient is informed that more uncomfortable and embarrassing tests are necessary, tears of self-pity may spill over. At the same time, through the tears, the patient may apologize, saying, "I know I shouldn't, but I can't help it. Usually I don't cry. I don't know why I am crying now."

Even as illness revives or produces childlike characteristics, in some cases, illness also represses mature reactions that have characterized the life before the illness. Frequently this is seen in the ill person's inability to "hear" what the physician is saying. Why do such a large percentage of those with breast cancer delay three months after noticing a lump before going to a doctor? Why do so many men persist in attributing chest pains to indigestion? This refusal to face reality and listen to the truth makes it hard, not only for the ill one, but for those who love them and visit them.

I recall, still with amazement, an experience I had. A friend phoned from the hospital. "The doctor has just told us I have cancer," she said, her voice breaking.

I answered stupidly, "Oh, no!"

Her only response was loud weeping.

"I'll be right over," I said.

But it took time to get someone to look after the children. When I arrived at the hospital, my friend was cheerful. She would be going home in a couple of days, she said. Her ailment was not serious, and she soon would be well again. I stood speechless. My friend never wavered from her position that she was not seriously ill until the day before her death a few months later.

We ask, "How can this be?" Perhaps it will help if we recall how close truth and fantasy are for children. Who of us cannot recall fantastic things we believed in thoroughly when we were children and the wishful thinking we did. I can recall telling my playmates I had wings in my drawer at home. I could put them on and fly, I said. I really believed I would be able to do so—if only I could find them!

So it will help us if we remember that the dependent state illness forces on us can produce unexpected reversions to childlike behavior. Living in an unreal world and not hearing what doctors are saying may be one way we revert.

Illness can make us preoccupied, absentminded, or forgetful too. The forgetfulness can persist through the period of recuperation. We may leave keys or wallet in stores or restaurants. In the process of making a cake we may not be able to recall whether or not we put in the baking powder.

Not infrequently bank accounts also get messed up.

How can we handle all of these strange things that are happening to us?

First of all, it will help both our families and us if we know beforehand what changes can take place. Then when the changes begin to happen, we need not be overly concerned but can realize these personality changes are just part of being ill and are temporary.

Sharing concerns with others also is helpful. We can tell our doctor about our need to have one specific person to whom we can talk.

When I became aware of the forgetfulness aspect of illness, I made notes of things I needed to remember. I did this especially if I was going in for surgery. If I put away an article in an unaccustomed place, I made note of that too.

If we find ourselves enjoying being sick and reluctant to become well because it will mean going back to the old work schedule, it will help to admit this—with a smile! And the next step is to phone our employer giving the date we hope to be able to return to work.

We also need to realize that the dependency illness enforces on us can have positive effects. Weakness and not feeling well makes us willing to relinquish work and home responsibilities. As we do this, we are better able to rest and relax—and this, in turn, facilitates healing.

Helps for Your Quiet Times with the Lord

We acquaint ourselves with what the Lord says

Read Mark 6:45-51. How would you describe the situation of

the disciples? What did Jesus do to help them? What message
do these verses have for you?

We reflect and meditate

Life is never so bad at its worst that it is impossible to live. It
is never so good at its best that it is easy to live.

GABRIEL HEATTER

Affliction comes to all of us, not to make us sad, but sober;
not to make us sorry, but wise; not to make us despondent, but
by its darkness to refresh us, as the night refreshes the day; not
to impoverish, but to enrich us, as the plough enriches the field,
to multiply our joy as the seed, by planting is multiplied a thou-
sandfold.   HENRY WARD BEECHER

We pray

Dark and cheerless is the morn unaccompanied by Thee;
Joyless is the day's return till Thy mercy's beams I see;
Till they inward light impart, glad my eyes, and warm my heart.

Visit then, this soul of mine; pierce the gloom of sin and grief;
Fill me, Radiancy divine, scatter all my unbelief,
More and more Thyself display, shining to the perfect day.

CHARLES WESLEY

What I Really Need Is...

It had been another cloudy, wet day outside, and a weepy, wet day inside for grandma, lying immobile from her stroke. Her grown granddaughter was sitting by her side.

"I'm no good any more, Mary," grandma said. "I'm not good for *anything*." And the tears overflowed again.

"Maybe you feel that way, grandma, but you're the only one who does," Mary said, smoothening her grandma's hair and holding her hand.

Mary understood that when we are ill we need to retain a sense of self-worth. Remaining in communication with others and finding ways to reach out are important also. Care-givers of the ill usually try to provide for the physical needs of the ill: proper food, adequate fluids, rest, physical activity, oxygen, and elimination, and all of these call for careful nursing care. Care-givers also express loving concern and try to help the ill one feel secure by maintaining order, sameness, and routine. But it is equally important that care-givers

35

provide also for the psychological comfort of the ill. All too often little thought is given to this.

Retaining a sense of self-worth or self-esteem is of primary importance, because illness cuts deeply into our sense of self-worth for a number of reasons.

Our culture places excessive importance on productivity. When we can no longer work or produce, a large portion of society is ready to cast us aside.

"I am unemployed now and apparently unemployable. The paper I owned is sold," a newspaper editor wrote. "My wife has had to go to work, and I draw Social Security."

It's disheartening when this happens. But placing prime importance on what we do is not really anything new. Even Jesus' disciples were caught up with this misconception. One day they came to Jesus all excited. They had been off on a preaching mission, and not only had they succeeded in turning people around, but they had healed the sick and cast out evil spirits. "Lord, even the demons submit to us in your name," they exclaimed (Luke 10:17).

Jesus listened, unimpressed. Then he said quietly, "Do not rejoice that the spirits submit to you, but rejoice that your names are written in heaven."

A man suffering from an impaired heart lamented that his social life had become almost nonexistent because he had energy for so little. He felt left out. Another man who had sustained hearing loss said social activities had become very difficult for him. He felt left out when he couldn't follow the conversation. When we feel left out, it's hard to continue to regard ourselves as being of value—or at least as being of as much value as before. We need to be reassured that we are of value simply because of what we *are*.

Norman Vincent Peale writes in his book *Dynamic Imaging,* "I believe the greatest health insurance a person can carry is to see himself, proudly and humbly, as a creation of God. God, who is infinitely gifted and infinitely wise, does not do bad work. If He created you in His image, and He did, that means His excellence, His craftsmanship are built into you."

However, it also helps when people notice any effort we are making and say things like: "I think it's wonderful you keep on with your therapy even when progress is so slow and painful." "I admire the way you've learned to discipline yourself." "You were kind to your crabby roommate." "You look attractive today." And if others don't affirm us in this way, there's nothing wrong in our affirming ourselves.

Disfigurement that may result from our illness also erodes our sense of self-esteem.

"Loss of physical attractiveness ate away at my confidence," Jeanne Crumley wrote. "My face was scabbed and scarred. I thought my wig was funny looking. My clothes hung loose since I had lost weight. I had to wear sunglasses all the time. Everyone else accepted all this as temporary, but still I felt unattractive. I did not always feel good, and thus I did not always act as warmly and graciously toward others as I wanted to. It just seemed as though I lacked the energy to reach out. Yet I still felt guilty and selfish. I think time was the single most important factor in working through these things and regaining self-esteem. Support from others helped too."

Minor disfigurements appear to cause more misery than major ones. Victims of severe burning, for example, often make remarkable adjustments while young people with acne can suffer acutely and withdraw. But it is possible to work one's way through and find a reasonably satisfactory solution. Being surrounded by family and friends who love us for what we are and don't fuss about the problem helps too.

So does deliberately doing what one fears to do. Loss of body beauty, in most cases, is only as important as we make it.

A number of doctors have noted also that nothing seems to help people accept and live with physical disfigurement more than a faith in God.

In addition to our need to retain a sense of self-worth, we have two other psychological needs: the need to remain in communication with others and the need to be able to reach out to others and give. Both of these needs are intertwined closely with self-esteem. When our self-esteem is low, we may ask if we have anything to give to others when we are ill. We forget the priceless gifts of the spirit which are always ours to give.

I remember, with gratitude, how much Bob Lange gave me. Bob eventually died from Lou Gehrig's disease, but during the three years he lingered, I received much from him that I could not have received if he had not been facing death. I know Bob helped me begin to face my own death. The dignity, calm, and courage with which he lived, knowing he was going to die soon, remain cherished memories in my heart, steadying and strengthening me. If God could enable Bob, God can enable me too when my turn comes, I reassure myself now when fluttering fears disturb.

Bob also helped me not to take myself too seriously. Just weeks before he died he used some of his meager energy to attend the Rose Bowl football game. I visited him a few days later. He was still exhausted from the effort. "But it was worth it," he said, smiling happily.

Knowing Bob's deep commitment to the Lord and seeing him balance this with pleasure has helped me maintain perspective.

Another friend, Marge van Dine, found a ministry in the

midst of her illness. The Lord Jesus had become a living bright reality to Marge during the early stages of her illness. She nourished that relationship through Bible study and prayer. As her disease progressed, Marge had to enter the hospital. There she was given a ministry of prayer. Noting her courage and serenity, nurses, interns, clerical staff and housekeepers came to her asking her to pray for them. If we really believe prayer is the mighty force we say, how could Marge have had a more powerful ministry?

But a ministry of reaching out like Bob's and Marge's becomes possible only when we are willing to communicate with people on more than a superficial level. Often we talk only about the weather, the news, and what's happening to people. When we confide something sad that has happened to someone we love, we go a little deeper. When we tell how this is making us feel, we are opening the door for a more intimate communication where soul can touch soul. Often, however, when we are well, our busy schedules prevent us from taking time to advance to the deeper levels. Illness enforces a "leisure" on us that enables us to converse more meaningfully with people, to give and to receive.

"At the time of sickness the mind is not cluttered," Dr. Gerald Strickler, professor of philosophy at California State University, Long Beach, observed. "Concerns about work are not as foremost or important. This enables one to enjoy, appreciate, and develop closer relationships. One can more easily accept and assimilate the 'reaching-outs' being offered us."

Communication, to become most intimate and helpful, should involve mutual sharing.

"I was fortunate in that I found it easy to be frank and open with my loved ones," a young person who overcame cancer said. "I really don't know for sure if my loved ones

39

were also open with me. Perhaps there was some effort to 'shield' me from their burdens."

In order to experience truly intimate communication we must be willing to let others know us as we really are. Illness offers us unique opportunities to do this. Illness, especially if it is serious, has a way of stripping us of sham and pretense. Not only is our body stripped naked time and time again for examination, but we feel our very selves standing naked—shivering a bit, to be sure, but seen for what we really are. This, however, can be tremendously liberating. "It's such a relief not to have to pretend at all any more," Bob said to me one day.

When we feel we no longer need to hide anything from the one with whom we are talking, we are set free to unburden our hearts of many things that may be troubling us. When this involves confession, the very deepest communion takes place. True confession is incredibly hard—hard for the one confessing and hard for the one listening to the confession. Dr. Paul Tournier tells of instances when he actually became ill after listening to confession. But such confession brings new life and energy coursing through the body, and it liberates the spirit.

"There's risk in openness, however," one noted. "If you choose to be honest about your feelings and thoughts, you also have to be prepared for all kinds of responses. Some things people say are bewildering. Some hurt. Not everyone understands."

"The effect of my illness on relationships with friends varied in response to their ability to deal with my illness," Jeanne Crumley wrote. "In most cases I found that if I was open to discuss it with them, they reciprocated, and we grew closer as a result. And I discovered that illness, like any crisis situation, enables one to broach topics that are not everyday topics of conversation."

Paul Hawkinson added that his wife, Linnea, was able to have more meaningful and satisfying conversations with visitors when they came one by one.

Usually we discover that when we have courage to be just what we are, people like our "true selves" better than our "pretend selves." Not always, however! It can be a shattering experience when one discovers that the person his or her friend had pretended to be was much nicer than the real person! When a husband or wife make this discovery, skilled professional counseling usually is needed, accompanied by a willingness on the part of both individuals to forgive, accept, and adapt. If this is not forthcoming, hitherto tolerable and even pleasant relationships may break down completely. That's the risk involved.

While intimate conversation is important, keeping in touch with people even on a lighter level is also important. Cards, letters, telephone calls, and visits *do* mean a lot to the sick one.

Usually it's the long-term or chronic illness or the drawn-out recuperation that presents problems. Paul Hawkinson solved it for Linnea. Once a month he sent a general letter to family and close friends, adding a personal note on each. As a result, Paul said, hardly a day passed that Linnea did not take a letter or card from the mailbox.

Sometimes illness can be of a nature that prevents talking. Following each stroke she had, my mother experienced more and more difficulty in speaking. Finally she learned that it was easier for her to form the sound of one letter than a whole word. Laboriously she would spell out her sentences to us. During those difficult days we were glad that communication isn't limited only to words--frustrating though it is when we want to say something and can't. Touch, looks, and humor become more important than ever.

Communication with others involves more than conversation, however. It also implies a willingness both to give and receive help. Sometimes it is hard for the ill one to welcome assistance. A young businessman told of his first reaction when he learned people were going to give him the proceeds of a baseball game. His oldest son had undergone open-heart surgery and another son had cancer. In addition, he had four other children to support.

"I was at a low in my spiritual life and said no to the idea of receiving help," this father said. "But then later I found Christ in a new and beautiful way. I was then able to say yes to the gift. Many more beautiful things were done for my family. I recall especially the day I went to the grocery store and realized I didn't have nearly enough money for what I needed. I closed my eyes and said, 'Lord, you'll just have to take over. I don't know what we'll do the next two weeks, but I know we'll be okay.' Less than two hours later friends backed up to our home with a car loaded with groceries. Talk about miracles!"

Members of a certain congregation discovered what happens when people cannot accept help. A member needed costly surgery that could be performed only in a distant city. Other members responded by sharing their resources to make the surgery possible. The woman's life was saved. Health was restored. But after the family returned home, they were never seen at church again. They were not able to accept the dependency illness imposed on them, necessitating their receiving help. They did not know how to receive help and still retain a sense of self-esteem.

In order that our hearts and minds can lie at rest, enabling healing to come and health to be restored, we need:

(1) to have our physical needs met, (2) to feel secure and cared for and cared about, (3) to relinquish our work, (4) to retain self-esteem, (5) to communicate with others, (6) to participate with others in giving and receiving, and (7) to reach out. Awareness of these needs can help us, our loved ones, and our care-givers. Then we can take definite action to see that these needs are being met adequately.

Helps for Your Quiet Times with the Lord

We acquaint ourselves with what the Lord says

Read Isaiah 41:6-7. Note how beautifully one person affirms another.

Read Isaiah 41:10, 13, 14, 17-18. Ponder these verses for comfort and reassurance.

We reflect and meditate

The ancient truth is that the health of the self comes, not by concentrating on self, but by such dedication to something outside the self, that self is thereby forgotten.

ELTON TRUEBLOOD

You are only really useless when you cease to want to be of use.   FRANCE PASTORELLE

Christ calls us to repentance, not so that we shall remain at this introspective stage, but so that, forgiven and set free, we can throw ourselves into action, and bring forth fruit, as he himself insists.   PAUL TOURNIER

We pray

What particular needs do you feel are not being met for you just now? Tell the Lord about them. Remember there isn't anything you need fear to tell him. Ask him to meet those needs. Then close your eyes and visualize those needs being met. Do this every time you pray for something: visualize the answer.

So You're Going to the Hospital?

I was in the hospital. On an extended trip to Asia I had picked up something that was causing uncontrollable diarrhea, nausea, abdominal pain, and weakness.

"We'll run some tests," the doctor said.

When I came back to my room after my first round of tests, a nurse presented me with Milk of Magnesia.

"What's that for?" I asked.

"More tests," was the only answer I got.

The purgative was effective. The running to the bathroom began. The psychological effect for me was bad. Days of uncontrollable diarrhea had weakened me. I had been greatly relieved when finally the diarrhea was stopped. Now it was being induced purposely. Apprehension and fear gripped me.

More purgatives followed that kept me scooting off to the bathroom all night. At 6 A.M. the nurse came with a quart of enema. I was so weak I burst into tears. The enema caused my already sore innards to cramp again. More running.

When I got down to the X-ray room, a preliminary scan

revealed I would need *another* enema! But first, they said, they'd do the kidney X-ray. I was taken aback. Nobody had told me I was to have a kidney X-ray. Why was I to have it?

What would it involve? A pint of an iodine solution injected into the vein of my arm, I was told. I was so exhausted and so tired of having needles stuck into me that I broke down and cried.

Why hadn't I been forewarned as to what tests would be performed and what the preparation for those tests would be? I asked. Then I could have prepared myself. And which of the several doctors who had seen me had ordered the kidney X-rays? I wanted to know.

The radiologist said he didn't know.

"That being the case," I said, "I will not submit until I know."

So they brought me back to my room. There I lay ignored by all for about two hours. The message I picked up was that I was being a "bad, uncooperative, difficult patient."

I finally succeeded in getting someone to call my doctor. He came, apologized for the confusion, explained the reason for the tests and what the tests would involve.

That afternoon when I reentered the X-ray room, the man in charge said sneeringly, "We were supposed to see you this morning. What happened? Turn chicken?"

I bit my tongue and prayed for control. Was it wrong, I asked evenly, if I wanted to know what was going to be done with me and who had ordered the tests?

His upper lip curled. "Did you have to know?" he asked. "Why get upset? When you go to a banquet, why not take the ham with the turkey?"

I pressed my lips together and said nothing.

"What's wrong?" he taunted. "Not talking, eh?"

46

I was seething inside.

It was late afternoon before I got back to my room. My doctor had assured me there would be no more purgatives. But there were. Plenty. The nurses told me about all the horrible things that would happen if I didn't take the purgatives. They refused to call my doctor. Evidently I was being a difficult patient again. Finally, completely worn out with resisting, I took the Milk of Magnesia and again ran all night.

The next day one of the young attendants from the X-ray department came to my room.

"How're you doin' today?" he asked. And then before I could answer he said, "It makes me so mad! It's so dehumanizing the way they treated you. I see it all the time. A person just isn't a person after he or she enters the hospital. The patient becomes an object for scientific observation, examination, and treatment. I hate it!"

But not only the health professionals were at fault. I should have asked more questions, insisted on more explicit answers, and made known my fears. As it was, I *did* feel like an object for scientific examination, and I did feel that I was treated as a person with not even a little gray matter in my head. I began to feel I was out of control, and when I picked up enough courage to assert myself I was rebuffed.

Just being admitted to a hospital can be upsetting. I would guess everyone's blood pressure and pulse goes up, even if one has been a patient before. If it's our first trip and if we haven't visited sick people in hospitals—wow! And for those for whom the hospital *is* a familiar place, the place itself calls forth memories. If the past experiences have been good, one feels reassured. However, if past experiences recall pain, loneliness, anxiety, apprehension, and sorrow, one cannot help but sigh, at least inwardly. Yes, being admitted to a

47

hospital is upsetting. People for whom the hospital is a familiar workaday world have difficulty understanding how upsetting it can be.

Another major threat to the patient is the loss of personhood. Somehow I seem to become a different person when I am admitted as a patient. I lose my identity, and it's always disturbing to lose one's identity. Illness has a way of leveling all of us. There's no status, class, professional or vocational association remaining. We're all just human beings, garbed in hospital gowns that make us feel like inmates. The band around our wrists with names and numbers identifies us.

"I'm not a person with a name anymore," a 17-year-old complained to me recently as he lay in the hospital. "My number on this band is checked every time they bring me medication. But who looks at me and knows who I am and calls me by name? Not many!"

Even the way the clergy approach us can either rob us of our sense of personhood or give us a sense of participation.

I recall a statement my mother made once when she was hospitalized. It had been our practice to have a time of Bible reading and prayer together every day when I came. This one day I greeted mother with, "We better have our prayer time first thing today. Yesterday we didn't get to it at all."

My dear mother, who usually treasured that time, gave a little snort. "I don't think I really need it today," she said candidly. "I've had four different preachers in here *praying over me.*"

A friend, back from an overseas trip, came down with malaria. "I became Exhibit A," he said. "I was the first malaria case they had had in that hospital. All the doctors and interns had to come and look at me."

It's difficult not to react to that kind of gawking. My grandfather did once. He dismissed himself and walked out of the hospital. "It's my body," he stormed. "I should be able to have a little to say about who looks at it."

Grandpa's action wasn't the wisest or the one always to be followed, but he did have a point. All of us want to be considered persons, not objects.

When we become ill, we lose our independence to a large degree. When we enter the hospital, we lose even more. We come under the control of others. During an examination we sit, stand, cough, don't cough, breathe, don't breathe, bend, or stretch at the direction of another. The hospital dictates when we shall eat, what we shall eat, when we shower, take walks, go to sleep, have visitors. On and on it goes. We no longer are in control. We are told what to do and what not to do. We begin to feel that we are being treated more like children than adults. Some of it seems so senseless.

On one occasion before surgery I volunteered to walk to the operating room. I had had no sedative and was clearheaded, cheerful, and feeling fine. The hospital attendants were horrified. I wasn't even allowed to hop out of bed and onto the gurney to be wheeled down the hall. Instead I had to shift myself awkwardly from bed to gurney. Ridiculous!

A friend, who had had a similar experience, noted in her journal, "More X-rays. Thought I had exhausted their repertoire. The orderly brought a *stretcher* for me! I asked him if I should dictate my will!"

The same friend asked for an aspirin one day. "It was a mistake," she said. "They had to make a federal case of it."

I remember my mother being refused the comfort of Mentholatum, which she had used all her life, on her chapped lips because "it hasn't been ordered."

When we discover that hospital rules are inflexible, we begin to feel we're under the domineering thumb of a parent again. It's hard not to feel resentful. Some of the feelings we had when we were adolescents begin to resurface. In the process of growing up we had developed our distinctiveness as individuals by expressing our independent thoughts and wishes. It was necessary then to learn to separate ourselves from Mom and Dad and become "our own persons." Now we feel we're under their authority again—in a slightly different form—and as we lose our independence, we also feel our identities beginning to slip away.

The nonchalance with which people walk in and out of our "bedroom" when we are in the hospital also robs us both of a sense of privacy and control. Following a stroke that immobilized her, my mother lay in the hospital. When I came one day she was giggling. A senile patient had wandered into her room and had drunk her orange juice, she said.

The isolation sickness imposes on us can be difficult to handle too. Just being unable to go to work or to church or to mingle with our friends isolates us. When we are admitted to the hospital, we are isolated even more. The hospital may be a distance away. Visiting hours are only at certain times. And for many people a hospital is such a threat that they cannot bring themselves to enter one, even though they may wish to visit an ill friend.

"I can't stand the smell," one says.

"I can't stand seeing people sick," another says.

"All I can think about is death. It's so morbid!" another insists.

Although most patients walk out of hospitals alive these days, sickness is a powerful reminder of our fragility and the certainty that one day all of us will die. Many people refuse to think about death, and so they will not come close to any suggestion of the body's deterioration—whether found in hospital or rest home.

But it isn't only being physically removed from people that isolates us. When we become ill, we become different from other people. People treat us differently too. And whenever we become "different" or are treated differently, it can produce a profound sense of loneliness. We want to be part of the crowd, but illness doesn't let us remain part of our old crowd. True, we become part of another crowd, but we're not too impressed with that crowd when we hear them moaning and groaning and see them lying almost "out-of-it" on their beds. So the cutting-off from our normal circle of friends and colleagues that we experience when we become ill can be hard to handle.

Sometimes the nature of our illness or treatment imposes severe isolation on us. Ione Johnson tells of her experience. "After two weeks of radium therapy every day the radiologist said I would be going in the hospital for a radium implant. That would last 60 hours. My daughters couldn't come to visit because they were of child-bearing age. My husband could come twice a day and stand at the door with a Geiger counter in his pocket. If it flared, he had to leave. His visits usually were two minutes long. The nurses and doctors stood on the other side of the large metal protective shield by my bed.

"Settled for the test, I reached first for my Bible. To my surprise I couldn't hold it. It was too heavy. I couldn't move, couldn't sit up, couldn't turn over. I was expected to remain in one position for 60 hours. Meals were brought in. I ate with my fingers, because I couldn't hold a fork. My daughters called on the phone, but I had to ask them not to call. It was almost impossible for me to grope around to reach the phone and talk. All my strength left me, and I couldn't move. The time was interminably long."

I experienced isolation during a case of pneumonia feared

to be highly contagious because four in our family had come down with it. I was put, not only in isolation, but in a steam tent. The inside fogged up, so I couldn't see the TV. My glasses fogged, so I couldn't read. The hissing sound interfered with listening to the radio. I had no phone. Because of all the hassle of gowning for isolation, the nurses' visits were infrequent. I soon discovered how unskilled I was in the practice of meditation!

How can we handle these threats?

Isolation and the loss of our sense of personhood and our independence may loom like formidable opponents. But instead we need to understand that what we view as threats, the hospital staff views as helps necessary so we can recover.

We complain that the objectivity with which the doctors and hospital staff treat us makes us feel like "the patient in 340" or "the gall bladder case" rather than feeling like Millie Tengbom or Judy Collins or whomever.

The care-givers protest: "We have to maintain a certain sense of objectivity or we wouldn't be able to carry on day after day."

And they are right. We need to understand that underneath their veneer of objectivity most health professionals are caring people. If they weren't they wouldn't be in the profession.

Our daughter worked for a while for a neurosurgeon who was given high-risk cases. She told of the times following an unsuccessful surgery when the surgeon would come back from the operating theater, go into his private office, and shut the door. Once, unaware that he was in his office, she entered to find him weeping.

"I have to cry," he said between sobs. "I feel so bad when my patient doesn't survive."

Yet that surgeon approaches his surgery in a seemingly detached manner. He may even joke and carry on a lighthearted conversation while he operates. But without that very objectivity he would not be able to continue to operate day after day.

At the same time health professionals are becoming more and more aware of how important it is to discover what the feelings of the patients are. Doctors and nurses are being urged to take time to talk with the patients and to encourage them to express their feelings.

The day after my traumatic experience with the kidney X-rays, a nurse I hadn't seen previously came on duty. She came into my room, introduced herself, pulled up a chair, sat down, and said, "Tell me what happened yesterday."

Evidently there had been some notations on the chart about how upset I had been. I told my story. She listened carefully. At the end she squeezed my hand and said, "Thank you for telling me this. I have learned much today."

Once after surgery I was left alone in the recovery room as I was struggling to regain consciousness. I say struggle, because it really was a struggle, and a most unpleasant experience. I wanted to become fully conscious but couldn't. *What if I don't?* I wondered and began to panic. *If only someone would stand by me, touch me, talk to me, reassure me!* I thought. I could hear the voices of young nurses off in a corner discussing their dates. I opened my mouth to call them but no sound came out. I wanted so much to get their attention! My helplessness distressed me greatly.

Later I shared the anguish I had felt with the nursing supervisor. A few hours later she appeared in my room with half a dozen students with her.

"I want you to tell these young women what you told me," she said.

I did.

"Now do you understand?" she asked the girls. "What we

53

try to tell you in the classroom isn't just theory. People really feel this way."

A friend who is a surgical nurse makes it a practice to arrive at the hospital an hour early. She visits the patients she will be caring for later in the operating room, answers questions, holds their hand, and reassures them. She greets them later at the door of the operating room and holds their hand until they slip into unconsciousness.

So health professionals are making efforts to regard patients as persons who are not only to be cared for but cared about. Not that it is easy to impress this on all. Hospitals still remain institutions of science, and in this discipline it's easy to slip into the practice of treating ailments and illnesses instead of treating people. And it will take time for youth growing up in a society that teaches us to focus on ourselves to forget themselves as they serve as professionals and learn to concentrate on the well-being of others.

We, as patients, can help too. In one sense, we have a responsibility to assume care for ourselves. If we feel we are being treated only as objects, we can remind the care-givers quietly and tactfully that we are persons, we have feelings and would like to be treated as persons. If after gentle reminders, the treatment does not improve, a wise move is to talk to our doctor and let him intervene for us.

Some hospitals provide patient representatives who interpret hospital philosophy, policies, procedures, and services to patients, their families, and guests and assure them of the hospital's desire to respond to their needs. Patient representatives also act on behalf of the patient in negotiating solutions to problems with hospital administration or departments. They implement those solutions and recommend alternate policies and procedures, if necessary, to improve future services to patients. And they follow up with the patient to ensure satisfaction. Some patient representatives even become involved in comforting families, obtaining absentee ballots for patients in major elections, helping patients fill out insurance forms, writing letters and thank-you notes for patients who are unable to do so, and making motel or hotel reservations for family or friends.

Many hospitals also have social workers, chaplains, or trained volunteers who can act as mediators between patients and the medical staff. In some hospitals you may have to ask to see them. But talking with someone who knows about illness, knows the hospital, and is a skilled listener can reassure and help.

Hospitals also are trying to ease the initial apprehension patients feel by projecting programs on the room television sets that welcome the patients and explain the hospital procedures.

Hospitals are trying to ease the feeling of isolation too by paintings hung on walls or wallpaper brightening them. Television sets and telephones put patients in touch with others. Windows in rooms look out on pleasant scenes when possible. One nursing home even allowed an isolated patient, who had spent all her life on the desert, to have her pet donkey tethered outside her window.

Volunteers come in with the morning paper and mail and later in the day wheel in carts with reading materials. Comfortable lounges allow opportunities for visits with friends or other patients.

Many hospitals offer the services of a chaplain, and a quiet chapel can become a private place to which the patient can slip away to pray. Prayer can help immensely to lessen one's feeling of isolation. We become more conscious of God's presence with us. Participation in the Lord's Supper also can ease one's sense of being alone.

Clara Carlson said she found quietly singing hymns relieved her sense of isolation.

Norman Vincent Peale tells of not being able to sleep and beginning to pray for everybody he could think of. "Actually, I must have prayed for five hundred people by name. By this time it was 6 A.M. and the night was gone. And all of a sudden I felt better than I had felt in a long time," he said.

Some have found it helpful to choose one Bible verse at a time and meditate on it. Some have read a story from the Gospels or listened to it on tape and then tried to imagine the scenes. They have tried to see the people, the expressions on their faces, the way they moved and walked. They have tried to imagine the tone of voice when people spoke. Others have reconstructed scenes from childhood, trying to fill in every detail. Others have sought to relive momentous days in their lives, savoring them again deeply. And when isolation involves complete separation from others, God is there with us, enabling us to endure.

Ione Johnson wrote of her isolation experience during radium implantation. "The 60 hours did pass," she said. "The doctor removed the long slender fillers that had been shot full of radium. It was almost midnight, but I was told that in the morning I could go home if I was able to walk. The nurse helped me to the shower. It was my first shower in a month and felt wonderful! I was walking on air. I could go home! 'You have done so much for me, Lord,' I said."

We also need to realize how important isolation is if we are to recover. Isolation removes us from home or place of work, making it easier to relinquish responsibilities and to worry less. This in itself helps us become well. And with our body's resistance lowered, we need to be protected from other infections. The isolation of a hospital protects us.

Helps for Your Quiet Times
with the Lord

We acquaint ourselves with what the Lord says

Read Isaiah 43:1-2. What message does God have for us in these verses?

We reflect and meditate

It is not miserable to be blind. It is miserable to be incapable of enduring blindness.   JOHN MILTON

Let's not pretend. No one *likes* pain or sickness or difficulty or a sense of darkness and being alone. But if we can accept it as part of life and hold on to God who, for the time, isn't there—apparently—we shall emerge eventually toughened and strengthened.   J. B. PHILLIPS

We pray

It is the morning hour,
And I do pause to pray
For needs on this new day.
For strength to meet each pain;
For patience without end;
For love, to love, as I am loved;
For forgiveness and peace of soul;
For hope that looks beyond the present;
For faith which knows no limit;
And for grace all sufficient.
I then give thanks for the rest,
And for the new day, in which I may
Serve and pray for others.
    CLIFFORD BOREN

Coping Skills

When middle-aged Olaf and Enid Olson (not their real names) went to bed July 3, 1970, they did not dream that within 24 hours both of Olaf's arms would be dangling uselessly by his side. Four months later, after weeks of agonizing pain, a 25-pound weight loss, and shoulder muscles so wasted away that Olaf's arms dropped out of the sockets, doctors at the Mayo Clinic made a diagnosis. Acute bilateral brachial plexitis, a rare nerve disease. The doctors knew of no medication or cure. They could not assure Olaf that he would be able to use his arms again.

"We went back to our motel room," Enid recalls. "The gloominess of that dark, rainy day matched the darkness within our souls. As I took out my Bible a tract fell onto the floor. I picked it up and read these words by F. B. Meyer:

"Their strength is to sit still" (Isaiah 30:7). Never act in panic. Force thyself into the quiet of thy closet until the pulse beats normally, and the scare has ceased to disturb. When thou art the most eager to act is the time when thou wilt make the most pitiable mistakes. Do not say in thine heart what thou wilt or wilt not do, but wait upon God until He makes known His way. So long as that way is hidden, it is clear there is no need of action, and that He accounts himself responsible for all the results of keeping thee where thou art.

"Being able to believe that God considered himself responsible for taking care of us helped me to accept the doctors' report," Enid said. "I told the Lord I would trust him. And I found peace."

How we cope when we are ill will be determined by a number of factors: our backgrounds, personalities, age, intelligence, emotional development, and religious beliefs and previous experiences with illness.

Olaf's natural disposition is patient and kindly. His illness was not the first hard blow he had encountered. In his early 20s his father had died. He ably had taken over the care of the family farm. Twenty years of riding out the frustrations and disappointments of farming had prepared him further. He had a strong, unquestioning faith in God from childhood and had nourished it carefully with a daily quiet time.

The type of illness will also affect how we cope. Olaf faced the possibility of not being able to work again. Still Enid and Olaf found strength and courage to take a day at a time, and faith kept hope lively.

Physiological problems also affect us. When Olaf's pain was intense, he could not think beyond his pain and wanted only to die. Enid insisted he think of his family's future. And concern for the ones he loved was able to overcome his wish to die.

Our environment also has a profound effect on how well

59

we cope. Olaf was surrounded by a strong, courageous wife, cheerful children willing to work and economize, a supportive extended family, and friends and neighbors eager to help. Olaf had a savings account, and the fact that the family could, to a large degree, live off their farm alleviated financial anxieties and gave Olaf a feeling of security. During his long months of therapy and recuperation, the lively chatter of his five youngsters and the merry laughter of his wife stimulated and encouraged him. He used his time to read, study his Bible, pray, and walk. He stayed alive.

Olaf admitted that to begin with he did not believe his illness was as serious as the doctor had said. Denial is a technique people sometimes use almost unconsciously. Sometimes, as in the case of a sudden traumatic accident or the sudden onset of a disease, it is a needed skill. Denial provides a cushion of time so we can prepare ourselves. However, if denial is persisted in, it prevents growth and enrichment both for ourselves and others.

The "give me time to handle this" reaction sometimes is manifested in going from doctor to doctor, hoping we'll get a more positive report. Getting a second or third evaluation is not wrong or even to be discouraged. Sometimes we can gain new information. Enid and Olaf did. And seeking the best possible medical help can relieve us later of feeling guilty because we didn't do everything possible. But if all the doctors concur on the diagnosis, the time comes when we must stop our running around and hear and believe what the doctors are saying, threatening though it may be.

Frequently following the initial reaction of not really wanting to believe the doctor's diagnosis comes a time of intense curiosity. We want to know everything.

The desire to know what really was wrong drove Olaf and

Enid to the Mayo Clinic where a diagnosis of the illness was made.

Support is immensely important in enabling recovery. The more support we get from family members, relatives, friends, colleagues, church, and community, the better chance we have for a quicker and more complete recovery. Strong support from many sources sustained Enid and Olaf.

They discovered, however, that friends and neighbors' support was most evident in the beginning. As is usually true, for the long haul the family proved to be the most faithful.

Families can also provide some help that friends cannot give as readily. Families can be honest and affirm acceptable behavior but also can confront the ill member if behavior is not acceptable. Usually a family embraces the same religious faith and values, and this also strengthens the sick one. And families can provide security and a restful, caring atmosphere.

Also in a good family a person is valued for what he or she *is*. The need to produce is not as necessary as it is in the working world. This helps the ill one retain a sense of self-worth.

Olaf and Enid learned to adapt. Because the children were going to school they could do only a certain amount of work. The cows had to be sold. Olaf knew also he couldn't expect the boys to do the work as well as he, and he accepted this. He also had to learn to watch Enid take over some of the farm work. None of this was easy.

Personally he had to accept Enid's help in dressing, bathing, and with the therapy exercises. She had to drive him wherever he needed to go.

Both of them had to learn to receive from others.

"People who are used to being in a position to give, find it hard to accept when they themselves need help. It is amazing how much we learn when roles are reversed, and we become receivers instead of givers," a pastor whose daughter was seriously ill wrote.

Learning to receive graciously, gratefully, without apology and rewarding the giver by the way we receive the gift is an art to be learned.

Anne Morrow Lindbergh, in *The Man Who Lived Twice: Edward Sheldon,* tells of her visits to a friend who was blind for 20 years:

> He gave abundantly; advice, encouragement, stimulus, criticism. . . . But he also allowed you to give to him. He knew how to receive so graciously that the gift was enhanced by its reception. It was the rarest pleasure to bring things to him, books one had found, passages of poetry or philosophy, comments on life by a soldier one had met in a train or by a child in a school bus. He took them all in eagerly. Warmed by his welcome, how beautiful became the things one brought him. So often one has the opposite experience, gifts shrivel under the critical gaze of the recipient. One is like a child running in from the beach with a jewel found in the retreating rim of the tide, only to have it fade to an ordinary stone on the dry palm of another. With Edward Sheldon everything became more beautiful in the light of his appreciation. Seashells became pearls; ordinary stones were jewels.

Olaf and Enid found that remembering all the ways God had been faithful to them in the past buoyed up their faith and trust. Enid said that, as the weeks passed, they began to feel God actually had been kind to them in letting the illness come. The experience was proving to be cleansing. Things had gone so well for them before, she said, that they had become quite self-sufficient. Now they were cast on God and forced to reassess their lives and reexamine their values.

"I had been complaining bitterly before about all the work a farm demands," she said. "Suddenly Olaf couldn't work at all. I was working harder than ever and discovering work was a great blessing.

"Probably because our family always had been so well and strong we never really had been able to understand why some people were sick so much, nor did we sympathize with them. Now we were discovering how fragile life is, how within a matter of hours a person can become more helpless than a baby. We discovered that, at heart, we had become profoundly grateful—grateful for all the gifts of the past, for any little improvement we saw, grateful for what we had left to build on, and grateful, most of all, that God loved us enough to chastise us.

As Olaf and Enid persisted in faith, hope, and therapy— painful though it was—Olaf's right arm and hand slowly became muscular and strong again. The left one remained weaker, and its use beyond a supportive role remains limited. But for a decade Olaf has been able to farm at full scale as he has adapted to his limitations and used mechanization to assist him.

In addition to Olaf and Enid, others also have found effective coping skills.

Many referred to the difference praising God made. "When Linnea became ill," her husband, Paul Hawkinson, said, "we decided to begin each day with praise. We thanked God for everything we could think of. When I left for work, we agreed to look for things for which we could thank God. It not only lightened our load, but it helped us enjoy each day."

Ione Johnson wrote of how much the Bible meant to her during her long painful months of treatment for cancer. "The morning I was to go for further X-rays I awakened at five,"

Ione said. "I thought back to an incident on a Saturday afternoon many years ago. Our daughter, Gretchen, was an avid fan of Maury Wills, famed for his base stealing with the Los Angeles Dodgers. Maury had written a book, *It Pays to Steal,* and was going to autograph his book at a shopping mall that afternoon. My husband had promised to take Gretchen, but interruptions delayed him. When they reached the mall, Maury had left. A sad little girl came home, but she hugged one consolation to her. 'I didn't get to see Maury, but I got his book!' she said. The book was second best, but a good second best.

"Strangely enough those words kept ringing in my ears. I lay there wondering if my cancer would be terminal. Would I meet the Master? I lay and thought about that for a long time. Then I thought, but if I don't get to see him now, I do have his book. That was important. It was second best. Seeing my Lord was first. But if I survived, I would have his book, and that would be enough. At peace, I went back to sleep. And the book sustained me through all the anxious months that followed."

Another friend spoke of the comfort received from the Lord's Supper. "It made Christ's presence with me tangible," he said.

Gathering information can dispel fears and help persons prepare themselves for what is ahead.

A woman who had a mastectomy said, "I wish someone had told me it's common afterwards to have crying spells and feel numbness in the arms. I had such problems sleeping too. Now I've discovered this is a common experience. Knowing this would have reassured me."

Sometimes we may feel that even our family doesn't quite understand what we are going through. Then the support from other groups can help us.

64

JoAnn McCoy, writing in *Guideposts,* told of how she suffered for years from agoraphobia, attacks of unreasonable, frantic fear of open spaces. When a psychotherapist told her that it was primarily a conditioned body response—a behavior disorder that could be unlearned—and not a mental illness, she was helped. But even more help came when she found others who were suffering in the same way. They began to meet together.

"How wonderful it is now," she notes, "to pick up the phone and call a sympathetic fellow sufferer when we feel distress or want to share a triumph."

Another emphasized the importance of being open about one's illness.

"It is important to be honest about how you feel, for without that no ministry is possible," a man wrote. "We can let others know how it is with us and still avoid false bravado, superficiality, or appeals for sympathy. To declare openly, 'I have cancer,' is what makes ministry from others possible. There is no guilt or shame attached to such an admission. Why try to hide it?"

A Christian doctor, writing of his illness, said he learned to be frank and honest with God too. He also refused to regard illness as being "laid aside." And, he said, it helped to know he didn't have to feel like a failure just because he had some inner spiritual struggles. "Instead I saw it as part of a growth process, and then I could welcome it," he said.

Struggling with the question as to why his little daughter had leukemia, James Claypool learned he should not be too quick in deciding that what had happened to them was only evil. He came to believe it was too early for them to know what the end result would be. He could think of examples of people who had experienced success, and yet later that very success exacted a very heavy toll. He said he also could think of some who had suffered traumatic incidents and yet through those very incidents life had become immeasurably enriched for them. So, he said in his book *Tracks of a Fellow Struggler,* he was learning to wait to see his daughter's illness in perspective.

Jeanne Crumley told of how it helped her to "turn outward." She had been finding it difficult not to be preoccupied constantly with her own illness. It had a way of creeping into every conversation, she said. But when she became aware of this, she deliberately began to reach out to other people, to inquire of them and become interested in what was happening to them. This brought relief.

If recuperation is drawn out or if our illness has left us with some impairment, we need to be reassured that we can take care of ourselves. Diabetics learn to give themselves injections. The one who has had a colostomy learns to take care of the apparatus and then forgets about the colostomy. The one who has had throat surgery because of cancer can learn to talk again, though it will be difficult. Those who have undergone heart surgery learn how to monitor themselves and recognize when they are getting too much exercise or not enough, when they are getting adequate rest or when the tensions are building up too much.

If the illness is of a terminal nature many have found realistic goal-setting helpful. Martha Blomquist did. "I want to live until all our children are on their own," she said. She did.

"I want to live until I can make a trip back East and visit all my relatives," she said. She did.

"I want to live until I hold a grandchild in my arms," she said. She did.

Eventually Martha did not see her last dream realized, but all her previous ones kept her eager and determined to live.

We could go on and on citing coping skills. My file is full of accounts of people who were able to live creatively with their illnesses and find in them opportunities for enrichment and growth. But they were able to do so because they were in living touch with Jesus Christ.

Dr. Paul Tournier, the Swiss psychiatrist who has seen so many people healed of seemingly incurable ailments, writes: "I feel that the deepest meaning of medicine is not in 'counseling,' but in leading the sick to a personal encounter with Jesus Christ, so that accepting Him they may discover a new quality of life, discern God's will for them and receive the supernatural strength they need in order to obey it."

Dr. Tournier said he constantly encouraged his patients to set aside time for reading the Bible and to follow that time by quiet meditation and listening to God in a spirit of expectancy. Then he encourages them to open their hearts freely to God. He said he explained to his patients that at first listening may be difficult. But, he assured them, if they persisted, they would hear God speaking to them. Then as they obeyed what they believed God was saying to them—always checking it out with the teachings of the Bible—they would find forgiveness and release.

Without doubt, finding our life, hope, and strength in Jesus Christ is the most effective coping skill of all.

Helps for Your Quiet Times
with the Lord

We acquaint ourselves with what the Lord says

Read Phil. 4:13. Paul was in jail when he wrote this. He did not know if the sentence of death would be pronounced for him or not. Yet in this difficult situation he was able to make this

declaration. Memorize this verse. Repeat it whenever you begin
to wonder if you can cope.

We reflect and meditate

Affliction . . . does not bereave of hope, but recruits hope. For
affliction compels the person mercilessly to let go of everything
else that he may learn to grasp the eternal and hang on to the
eternal.   SOREN KIERKEGAARD

The trouble the Artist takes to use every kind of discipline
that evil brings into life as a means of purifying our character,
though intolerable to us at the time, is a tremendous compliment,
and when we cry out to be left alone, we are asking for less care,
not more care, for less love, not more love.

LESLIE WEATHERHEAD

We pray

Drop Thy still dews of quietness,
Till all our strivings cease;
Take from our souls the strain and stress,
And let our ordered lives confess
The beauty of Thy peace.
    JOHN GREENLEAF WHITTIER

I Hurt!

One night at 10:30 my hand encountered a mass on my body. I phoned my doctor the next morning.

"Surgery," he said after examining me.

I felt my lips beginning to quiver and my eyes stinging. I was just beginning to feel good after four months of various illnesses—and now this!

"Look," my doctor said. "This isn't an emergency. Come back in a month."

My feet dragged me out to the parking lot. The bright sunshine mocked me.

It's not the surgery I fear, I told myself. *It's the horrible back pain after surgery.*

A congenital malformation in my lower spine caused my body to scream out in angry protest after it had been stretched out on the operating table. A shot of morphine would make the pain bearable for two hours. Then it would rear its angry head again, causing me to writhe on my bed, wet with perspiration, pleading for another shot. The last time I had had foot surgery my surgeon had come into my room.

"How are the feet?" he asked.

"I don't know."

"What do you mean, you don't know?" His voice was sharp.

"My back hurts so bad I can't feel my feet."

My doctor told me later that alarmed him because foot surgery usually is very painful. He reckoned if I wasn't feeling pain in my feet, my back pain must really be bad. It was.

Now faced with another surgery, all the memories of past pain came surging back. Anxiety grew. I tried to dispel it by reading my Bible and by praying. And I tried to tell myself I had nothing to fear, and that I was not afraid. It was a lie, of course. I *was* afraid. And as Montaigne stated: "He who fears he will suffer, already suffers because of his fear."

My subconscious mind tried to make me face reality. I began to dream terrifying dreams that left me gripped with even more fear.

The days passed relentlessly. Then two things happened.

The morning before entering the hospital I drove to a friend's house to return an article. As we talked we carefully skirted the concerns that lay most heavily on our hearts, but then one by one they began to spill out. Suddenly my fear and anxiety lay there too, bare and quivering.

My friend was on her knees in front of me instantly, her arms holding me close as she prayed. Then later, with both of us calmed, she said, "Once when I was living with fear, a friend pointed out that fear is an emotion of the future."

Of course! It was not a new thought. Our loving Lord had said it in slightly different words once when his disciples were troubled. "Do not worry about tomorrow, for tomorrow will worry about itself. Each day has enough trouble of its own" (Matt. 6:34). But I needed to hear those words again.

As I walked out to my car, I noticed how fresh the spring day was. I became conscious that my body was feeling charged with more energy than it had for months. As I drove home, I began to sing softly. Today was God's precious gift to me. And today was not only bearable; it was beautiful.

That night I said to my husband, "Why don't we pray that my back pain will be lessened?"

I had been hesitant to pray for any deliverance before. Twenty-six years earlier our second little son had been born prematurely with his lungs not fully developed. At that time I had prayed stubbornly that God would touch and heal him. When instead he died (our first son too had died), the lights went out for me. Ever since I had been careful not to pray for miracles. I didn't want to risk getting hurt again. Better to suffer through something, I thought, than to be disappointed again. But now my body seemed to be telling me it didn't want to hurt again, and I couldn't control my fear. And to pray that God would lessen my pain seemed right.

That night I slept peacefully. The mockingbird in our backyard, trilling his repertoire, awakened me in the morning. I found his song echoing in my heart.

In the afternoon I entered the hospital. The upbeat spirit continued through that day and greeted me the next morning, the day of my surgery. Even though my surgery was delayed until 2 P.M., still peace prevailed. No preliminary tranquilizer or sedative was given—nor needed.

I explained my previous back problems to the anesthesiologist, however. He listened sympathetically and promised to make me as comfortable as he could. At the same time he cautioned me that almost every patient put in this particular position experienced post-operative pain. However, he reassured me they would do everything they could to control my pain. I need not be fearful.

Hours later I awakened sleepily. Cautiously I inquired of my body. There was *no* pain. Carefully I moved in bed. No pain. No pain at all.

That night the nurses hovered over me because my blood pressure lowered and the intravenous needle kept slipping out of my veins. But still no pain.

Lying on my bed the days that followed and gazing out the hospital window at the trees and blue sky and fluffy white clouds, I thought about my experience. I wondered at the close connection between anxiety, fear, and pain. I recognized also that being set free from fear had been for me a miracle. Too many previous experiences of excruciating pain had imprinted themselves indelibly on my memory. Those memories victimized me, and fear held me captive.

I had been wary of praying for healing. But somehow, facing this surgery, I had been so unable to cope with my fear that I had felt the only thing I could do in my helplessness was cast myself on the Lord.

Now looking back from the perspective of a few years I realize how aptly my experience portrayed what doctors have discovered. The amount of pain we feel is affected by a number of things: the site and degree of the area injured or suffering, the sensitivity of our nerve endings or our pain threshold, how anxious we are, our previous experience with pain. Have we known times when pain has been unbearably painful and hard to control? What is our attitude to pain? Do we resent it? Become angry? Feel frustrated? Anxiety plus fear, plus guilt, plus frustration all equal more and more pain. What is our general health? Have we been sick for a long time? Are we in a weakened condition and worn out? What is the attitude of our family or friends? Are they anxious? Do they pour sympathy and pity all over us? Reassure us? Support us?

Some pain, unquestionably, has its roots in physical problems. However, some pain cannot be traced to a physical source. Physicians readily admit this. They do not deny the pain, but they emphasize that pain occurs in a milieu of relationships with other people. Many factors affect the degree and the possibility of finding relief. But resorting to surgery, as is commonly done, may not remedy the situation and may even exaggerate it. Surgery always should be the last option.

In his book *Pain: A Personal Experience* Dr. J. Blair Pace suggests that the services of a trusted, qualified psychologist or psychiatrist be considered before surgery if the cause of chronic pain is unidentifiable. The Minnesota Multiphasic Personality Inventory, he believes, may tell the doctor more than X-rays, does not cost more, and may get the suffering one on the road to recovery.

There are a few who insist on making pain a career. They go from doctor to doctor and from surgery to surgery. Had the man who had been lying by the pool of Bethesda for 38 years made a career out of his pain? "When Jesus saw him lying there and learned that he had been in this condition for a long time, he asked him, 'Do you *want* to get well?'" (John 5:6).

Those suffering chronic pain, the cause of which cannot be discovered, may be helped by facing and trying to answer honestly a few questions: Do you really want to be made well? Will you work with others to become well? What would you be doing if you did not have pain? How would you feel about this? What will you lose if you give up your pain? What can you do for yourself to achieve your goals?

This is not to imply, however, that if the cause of pain

has not been discovered yet, the pain has only psychological roots. Sometimes it takes a long time for doctors to discover the cause.

What can we do to transcend pain besides using prescribed medication?

In some instances heat, massage, and exercise bring relief. So can having someone to talk to or deliberately doing something for others. Some, confined to their beds, have used their imagination to redecorate a room, plan trips, lay out gardens, envision floor plans for dream homes, recall childhood scenes or joyous experiences. Others find listening to music to be healing. Sometimes feeling free to give vocal and physical expression to pain helps.

"I found rocking back and forth helped," one wrote. "And sometimes I even screamed and found, to my surprise, that helped."

Losing one's self in a mystery or a humorous book can distract. Norman Cousins, editor of the *Saturday Review,* said he had found that one "good belly laugh" a day did him immense good.

Listening to the Word of God from a tape recording has comforted many. And without question, when pain is so severe that our vision is distorted and we are nauseated and sick through and through and wish we could die, God alone is our only source of help. We begin to learn the meaning of endurance, and we no longer speak disparagingly about a "pie-in-the-sky" theology. We appreciate in a new way our Christian hope for a pain-free life after death.

However, with pain an unavoidable part of life, perhaps the most critical need we have is to reexamine our attitude toward pain and suffering.

Our culture tells us pain is an enemy to be obliterated. We have "ouchless" Band-Aids, aspirin for headaches, pep pills for tiredness, and sleeping pills for insomnia. We have silicone injections for inadequate bosoms, and face-lifts, toupees, wigs, and hair dyes to allay the signs of aging. Librium and Valium, the tranquilizer twins, have become the greatest financial success stories in the history of drugs. In recent years Valium has been the most often prescribed drug, and Librium has been number four. The annual sales volume of these two drugs has been enough to provide every adult and child in the United States with 20 pills yearly.

"Americans are probably the most pain-conscious people on earth," Norman Cousins believes. "For years we have had it drummed into us—in print, on the radio, over television, in everyday conversation—any hint of pain is to be banished as though it were the ultimate enemy."

This unrealistic approach to pain, suffering, and death may be one of the gravest problems that not only we as individuals, but we as a nation, face. Grave because when we are unrealistic about suffering, we are left confused about what to do when it does accost us. Grave because it may affect our moral decisions. Grave because we are missing out on the positive aspects of suffering. We are not allowing suffering to cleanse, enrich, and motivate us.

While we should be grateful for the relieving and comforting aspects of medical drugs and competent care, it is wise to remember that constantly eliminating and blocking out pain may cause us to expect life to deal only the good cards to us. Then we will be surprised and dismayed by pain or discomfort when they come.

In contrast I remember the remark of a venerable old Scottish missionary I knew in India. We were traveling to a conference on the third-class coach of a train. Third-class coaches boasted only hard, wooden-slatted benches that ran the length of the coach and a backless wooden bench in the middle. The windows had no glass, only iron bars. Through the bars drifted soot and dust, but even more uncomfortable were the chilling night winds off the Himalayas as our route ran parallel to those snow and glacier-covered mountains.

During our first night I sat shivering under the blanket I had wrapped around me. "Daddy Duncan" (as we affectionately called our friend) huddled beneath his woolen gray overcoat.

"Mr. Duncan, are you comfortable?" I asked.

The gray heap stirred; the sloping bald head emerged. Two faded-blue, birdlike eyes regarded me briefly.

"Comfortable?" he snorted. "I didn't know I was supposed to be!" And he disappeared under his coat again.

The comforts of life today have conditioned us to expect ease and freedom from pain. We parents also tend to shield and protect our children from pain.

Years ago people were more familiar with pain and suffering. Babies were born and people died at home. My grandmother was the community "mortician," loved by her neighbors because she was willing to go to their homes to perform this service of love.

Also during the early years of our country most people lived on farms. They knew the frustrations of having to adapt to unpredictable weather, animal sickness, pests, and trouble on every hand. They knew that pain and suffering and death are part of the fabric of life—that fruit, vegetables, animals, fowl, and fish have to die in order that people might live. They knew that the milk which they drank was theirs only because every year cows gave birth, in pain, to baby calves. Today, in our urban world, we are far removed from our sources.

Also, how strange it is that although our Christian faith has become possible only because of pain, we should be so surprised by the presence of pain in the world. Or have we, even in our teaching of the Christian faith, tried to ignore or gloss over Christ's physical sufferings?

We hear few sermons preached on the physical pains of Jesus. Perhaps even in this area we want to avoid mention of suffering.

Is it significant also that in our symbols we seem to avoid symbols of suffering and pain? The cross is empty. Rightly so, to be sure, and yet by portraying it empty we strip it of its pain.

In many of our church buildings we also have exchanged the altar, the symbol of suffering, for the table. The table is a comfortable symbol. It reminds us of home, of food and drink, of laughter and good times, of games and relaxation, of being part of the group around it and of being loved.

The altar is an unfamiliar figure to us. We have never heard the bleating of animals being slaughtered. I became aware of this on a trip to Israel. We were in Bethany, walking down a lane on our way back from a visit to a tomb, allegedly the one where Lazarus had been laid. I heard distressed bleating and peered over a wall. There in a courtyard a man was chopping the heads off goats. Blood ran freely. The sight sickened me. And then I thought of what the temple at Jerusalem must have looked like when sacrifices were offered. I wondered also if seeing animals killed as an offering for sin did not impress on people the awful seriousness of sin—something we seem scarcely able to grasp these days, for even in our worship our symbols may remove us from the sacrificial altar.

But only through the physical suffering, pain, and death of Christ has salvation come to us. Our reunion with God has been possible only because Christ was willing to endure pain.

Strange then, isn't it, that when pain has played such a

major and central role in our faith, we who claim to be Christ's followers should expect to be exempt from pain?

There is yet another aspect of suffering which I confess I do not understand. For years I had considered pain only as the enemy, the invader. But when I read the biographies and writings of some of the mystic saints of old I found myself forced to rethink my views on pain. Many of these men and women received in their bodies the *stigmata,* the wounds identical to those that marred the body of our crucified Lord. With the wounds came pain.

Catherine of Siena prayed she would be spared the marks because she did not want people to venerate her. But the pain was given, pain so severe that she wrote, "unless the Lord works a new miracle, it does not seem possible that the life of my body can endure such agony."

Pain given by God? I am puzzled by this. If so, then why?

A dearly loved and respected friend, who experienced slow death from cancer that spread into the bones, believed pain had been given to him by God for a specific reason.

"All my life I have felt compassion for all who have prayed for healing but not experienced it," he said to me some weeks before his death. "So when the doctors told me I had cancer, I accepted it as a commission from God. I felt I was being given an opportunity to show how we can endure pain with courage as we appropriate God's grace and help. I asked my friends not to pray that I would be healed. I recalled to them Jesus' words that blindness had come to a man in order that God might receive glory through it. I told them I wanted God to get glory through my illness. I use the pain medication my doctor prescribes for me, but it cannot block out all the pain which sometimes is very severe. But though my body pains me, my spirit rejoices in God, my Savior. For when I accepted my illness as a commission from him, I experienced a baptism of joy that has not left me all these many long months.

Our friend, who had had a long, fruitful ministry, continued to teach and preach on Sundays. When he spent the coldest winter months in the South he preached at the mobile-home court where he stayed. Word spread, and many people came from a distance, filling the hall that holds over 200, and 200 more stood or sat outside. Without question God was glorified through our friend's illness and pain.

Illness, pain, and disability need not impoverish us. Received rightly, pain can open to us doors of triumph, wholeness, and ministry that probably would not be possible any other way.

Helps for Your Quiet Times with the Lord

We acquaint ourselves with what the Lord says

For comfort read Revelation 21:1-4; 2 Corinthians 11:16—12:10; Philippians 1:29-30; 2 Timothy 2:3; Hebrews 12:1-15; and 1 Peter 2:21.

We reflect and meditate

Sickness teaches that activity of service is not the only way in which God is glorified. In our bearing suffering God is also glorified.   HORATIUS BONAR

The Son of God suffered unto death, not that people might not suffer, but that their sufferings might be like His.

GEORGE MACDONALD

79

In suffering we enter the depths; we are at the heart of things; we are near to where Christ was on the cross.

HENRI NOUWEN

We pray

Lord! a whole long day of pain now at last is o'er;
Darkness bringing weary strain comes to me once more.
Round me falls the evening gloom; sights and sounds all cease;
But within this narrow room night will bring no peace.

Come then, Jesus! o'er me bend, and my spirit cheer;
From all faithless thoughts defend, let me feel Thee near.
Then if I must wake or weep all the long night through,
Thou the watch with me wilt keep, Friend and Guardian true!
   LYRA GERMANICA

Machines– Friends or Foes?

A few years ago a nurse who worked in a cardiac care unit wondered if her career was going to come to an abrupt end. Her heart was giving her serious problems.

"You need a pacemaker," her doctor said.

She stalled, then finally agreed. The pacemaker was placed back of her breast tissue. It made no obvious difference in her appearance. At first she experienced some pain when she moved her arm or shoulder or twisted her body, but that too disappeared. To begin with she felt profound relief and gratitude as she knew death from an ailing heart was no longer imminent. Making friends with the machine inside her took a little longer. Little by little, though, as she learned to trust it, her anxiety eased.

"My level of activity still is limited," she says, "but not my scope. I swim, mow my lawn, paint my house, and work in nursing. We who are pacemaker patients can live normal productive lives if we follow a few rules and regulations:

exercise, daily pulse taking, periodic check-ups, and just generally taking care of ourselves."

Machines and artificial systems are offering more and more people extended years of productive living. People who have undergone colostomies learn to take care of themselves and rejoin life. Colostomy mutual aid clubs offer tips, encouragement, and support.

Those who need dialysis for survival face more complex problems. In many cases, before beginning treatment they have been so ill they have been virtually invalids. Once they begin treatment, others expect them to rejoin life and seek employment. To begin with, some are overjoyed. But as time goes on, joy fades as they have to spend 20-30 hours a week on a machine, preceded by strict dietary and fluid restrictions. This constantly interrupts job and family schedules. Bills pile up. The temptation comes to feel angry because one's body cannot function normally. Irritability and crabbiness upset the family further.

But if the persons can survive this difficult period of adjustment, there is hope for a continuing, meaningful life. Acceptance of one's limitations and the possibility of occasionally not feeling well is crucial. Some, whose work permits them to do so, learn how to carry on with letter dictation and phone calls even when on the dialysis machines.

Significantly many doctors recognize that Christian faith, more than anything else, appears to help people make this adjustment. Second in importance is the loving, encouraging, affirmative support of family and friends.

When one can be reasonably sure that machines will provide for a productive and even enjoyable lengthened life, the question of whether to use machines does not involve agonizing decisions. But what if one's condition worsens to the point that one can stay alive—though perhaps do little more than that—only if hooked up to machines? Do the machines then become friends or foes, burdens or vehicles of opportunity for prolonged life?

As long as physicians hold out hope for life being able to continue later without machines, the decision is not difficult. Often, however, physicians cannot be sure. And perhaps it is always a mistake to say any specific period of time is left for the patient. In situations like these who makes the decision?

Perhaps a preliminary question needs to be asked. *When* is the decision to be made? Some argue one cannot make the decision until one is faced with a definite situation.

But at the same time, if one waits until one is actually confronted with a specific situation, emotions can interfere with good judgment. Far better if we all could reflect on the subject while still well and then express to each other our personal wishes. A chaplain at a large hospital observed that whenever people, while still well and before a crisis, had discussed thoroughly the artificial prolongation of life, the decisions at the hospital were much easier. He emphasized also the value of the "living will" or preferences that had been expressed in personal handwriting. "It will save much grief and heartache," he declared.

Perhaps the best procedure to follow is to study beforehand what our Christian faith has to say about life and death, reflect on what it means to us personally, express tentative choices, and then be open to final decisions as we face actual situations.

Respect for each individual implies we consider the person's expressed preference. It follows, then, that we should be truthful in all we say to the ill person and to the immediate members of the patient's family. Often, however, it is wise to impart the facts one by one, allowing time for the recipients to prepare themselves to hear the ultimate.

Nor do we abandon hope after we have been told death appears inevitable. Hope has many facets. Hope does not mean only assurance that life will continue for many years. A remission of a few weeks or years can be held out as hope. Relief from pain can also be an offer of hope.

But who makes the decision when decisions have to be made? Usually the wisest decisions can be made when several people participate: the ill person, the family, the doctor, other medical staff, the hospital chaplain or family pastor. If the ill person is incapable of or has not expressed an opinion, the situation becomes more difficult. Some hospitals have a hospital ethics committee that can help those left with the decision making.

Occasionally difficult situations arise when the ill person, because of diminished mental ability, a distraught emotional state, or severe pain, is not capable of good judgment. When this happens, the presence of family, hospital staff and pastors becomes even more important. If decision making can be delayed, it is advisable to wait. If the ill person is begging to die, go slow. Sometimes—when, for example, pain is relieved in a few days—the patient no longer wants to die.

Sometimes a patient cannot evaluate fairly his or her chances for recovery if a certain treatment, painful though it may be, is followed. Nor can a child make as wise a decision as an adult. In such cases decisions need to be reached by others than the patient. The well-being of the ill person, however, must be carefully considered.

But what does one do when there is doubt as to whether or not the patient is irreversibly dying? Does one use a respirator then or administer cardiopulmonary resuscitation?

A general rule could be: "When in doubt, don't withhold," or, to put it positively, "When in doubt, treat."

Cancer patients frequently are given the option of choosing what form of treatment they wish. Some choose the treatment that holds some hope for a longer remission even though the effects of the treatment may be devastating. Others choose the shorter but less agonizing span. In this instance the preference of the patient is given priority.

In making the decision, however, the patient needs to remember that we don't "live unto ourselves and we don't die unto ourselves." Our decisions affect others. Sometimes it is possible to fight so desperately for life that we kill our loved ones in the attempt. Not infrequently, after a cancer patient has endured months of excruciating pain and unbelievable side effects from treatment only to die eventually, the surviving members of the family find themselves faced with problems of addiction to drugs or alcohol. It is very difficult to love a person, see that person suffer, and not overidentify with that loved one in his or her suffering to the point that to block out the pain we may resort to using measures that previously we never would have considered. If we are faced with having to help people in situations where they have become chemically dependent, we do well to remember Viktor Frankl's cautionary words: "No persons should judge unless they ask themselves in absolute honesty whether in a similar situation they might not have done the same."

Decisions regarding life and death are never easy. What appears to be a right decision at one time later may be regretted or viewed as a mistake. But God's forgiving grace and mercy covers all. He understands our human limitations far better than we and accepts and works within them. He is and remains a merciful God, slow to anger and abundant in loving-kindness.

Helps for Your Quiet Times with the Lord

We acquaint ourselves with what the Lord says

Read James 1:5-6; James 3:17; Isaiah 9:6.

We reflect and meditate

Courage does not come from an absence of fear, but from overcoming fear. A courageous person is one who goes ahead and does what he or she has to do *in spite of fear.*

What we need is courage to endure and willingness to let go and the sense to know when to do which.

We pray

For what do you need courage? Talk to the Lord about this. Open yourself to receive the strength he stands ready to give you. Pour out your heart to him. Ask for the wisdom he has promised to give.

Anxiety: the Mother of Knowledge

When doctors could not pinpoint the cause of Chin Young Petrusson's hemorrhaging, they suggested perhaps she had been taking too many aspirin. But something deep within Chin Young refused to be reassured. And then she had two strange experiences. She doesn't know whether to refer to them as dreams or visions—they really were neither.

Suddenly she saw herself in a building with the walls closing in on her. She cried out in terror. The building vanished, but in its place a huge black mass gathered overhead and then slowly dropped down on her, enveloping and smothering her. She struggled and cried out, and then realized the black mass had disappeared. She was lying on her hospital bed trembling violently. A strong sense of impending danger gripped her. She called for her doctor, related her experience, and said, "Something very serious is wrong with my body. We must find out what it is. Are there no other tests?"

Her doctor looked at her thoughtfully. "Yes," he said, "there is one. If you wish, we shall do it."

The test revealed cancer. So extensive was it that the surgeon later had to remove Chin Young's entire stomach.

Now many years later Chin Young recalls that incident with thanksgiving. "God was good to make me feel so anxious and worried," she says. "If I hadn't had those two frightening dreams or visions, I wouldn't have insisted on further tests, and I wouldn't be alive today."

Anxiety, if not ignored, can be the mother of knowledge.

Identifying the cause of our anxieties is the first step. What is making us anxious? Fear of pain? The possibility of the breakdown of family relationships because of the added stress of illness? The future welfare of our family? Bills? Uncertainty as to whether or not we shall be able to care for ourselves if recovery is not complete? Disfigurement?

Is there a practical way we can deal with these anxieties? Many have found the following procedure helpful.

1. Put in actual words what is troubling you. If a number of things are causing anxiety, give them a priority rating. Decide to deal with those that get the highest rating first.

2. Ask: Is there something I can do about what is worrying me? If so, what *can* I do? Find one or two friends or a pastor or a counselor with whom you can discuss this.

3. Decide on what definite steps you can take.

4. Act on what you decide.

5. Meet with your friends or counselor within a week or two weeks' time. Assess your progress. If the anxieties have not lessened, is there another course of action you should take?

6. Continue to follow this procedure.

But illness can present us with anxieties that are much deeper and more difficult to deal with. Illness always reminds us that we are mortal. Whenever we allow ourselves to think about the fact that one day we too will die, disturbing anxieties may agitate us. And this may happen in spite of the fact that we believe the Scriptures teach us, in one sense, that both death and life are part of God's created order.

If we refer to Genesis 2 and 3 we note a number of things. First of all, we note that God told Adam and Eve that they were not to eat of the tree of the knowledge of good and evil because in the day they did they would die. Was the death referred to physical death or spiritual death? It hardly would seem to be only physical death, for in reality Adam and Eve did not die "in the day that they ate."

But even if we believe that death is normal, as is birth, still there is an element in death that can be profoundly disturbing and anxiety-producing. The birth of a baby can be greeted with joy. Why? One of the reasons surely is that the adults welcoming the baby know life as a reality and know that life can offer many joys. Life is a known, not an unknown.

Death is different. The Bible teaches that life does not end with physical death. We are spiritual beings encased in physical bodies, and the spiritual aspect of our beings is eternal. There is a transcendency about human life. Something within us affirms this. Physical death is but the threshold over which we pass to enter the other dimension. But because it is a threshold over which few have passed and returned and about which we have no firsthand reports, the prospect of the experience can unsettle us. Jesus raised Lazarus from the dead. The Gospels record the fact that following Jesus' death some were resurrected. But all—including Jesus—have remained silent about the experience. Death and the life beyond remain a mystery. As Helmut Thielicke expressed it: "Death becomes a problem because it ends something unique and is something more and other than a natural process."

Death is a somber event. In one sense if we believed that

life ended with death, death perhaps would be easier to accept. There, of course, would be a certain poignant sadness about it, but there also would be a sense of finality about it. The unknown aspect of the life after death can be unsettling.

There are other aspects of life and death that may cause anxiety too. Paul Tillich believed that the dominant form of anxiety has varied from period to period. At the end of the Greek civilization, fate and death caused anxiety. At the time of the Reformation, it was guilt and condemnation. In our time he believed it is emptiness and meaninglessness.

I have asked myself, Is it meaninglessness that causes me anxiety? It may be for many, but my answer is no, no, no! Life has been full of meaning. Life has been rich. Indeed, even if there was no life beyond the grave, still life has been so good—in spite of all the evil it also has contained—that life would have been infinitely worthwhile.

I am not a fatalist either. Tillich says fatalism resulted when the Greek civilization crumbled. To be sure, some things result as a natural effect, but in many cases I can still control things. And even though at the end I shall not be able to stop death, still I am not a fatalist. I believe that God is in control, and that God can and does and will intervene in history—my own personal history and history as it concerns all.

But what about the guilt and condemnation which Tillich believed caused anxiety at the time of the Reformation? Guilt? Yes, I feel guilt. Condemnation? No. For I believe Jesus bore the guilt of my sin when he died and therefore there is now "no condemnation for those who are in Christ Jesus" (Rom. 8:1). I believe that God's offer of forgiveness and reconciliation is extended to all who will receive it. So while I experience guilt, I do not feel condemned, but forgiven.

At the same time I find that I cannot ignore the scriptural teachings on judgment, and this can occasion anxiety. Having had opportunities to teach, I cannot ignore verses like James 3:1: "Not many of you should presume to be teachers, my brothers, because you know that we who teach will be judged more strictly." Or Hebrews 9:27-28: "Just as man is destined to die once, and after that to face judgment. . . ." Or Romans 14:10: "We will all stand before God's judgment seat." Or 2 Corinthians 5:9-10: "So we make it our goal to please him, whether we are at home in the body or away from it. For we must all appear before the judgment seat of Christ, that each one may receive what is due him for the things done while in the body, whether good or bad."

I sometimes am troubled, for I know I have been selective as I have read God's Word. I have always been quick to underline and appropriate promises of forgiveness, help, and comfort. I have retained the right, however, to interpret or ignore other verses so they won't disturb me or make me too uncomfortable. I fear they might make too heavy demands on me if I took them seriously.

Take, for example, the inequality in our world. Fortunately or unfortunately, I have lived in lands and among a people of acute need. Shortly after I arrived in India the young child of a woman I knew choked to death. The worms with which that child was infected became so numerous they crawled up the throat and out of the mouth and asphyxiated the child.

When my colleague and I moved to a village to live, we could not sleep at night because the one surviving child of the family living in the shed in our backyard cried. He was cold and hungry.

When we lived in Africa, our youngest son's best friend

and dearly loved playmate died of complications following measles simply because he needed a tracheotomy and there was not 24-hour nursing care available for him. Had he been in the United States, he likely would not have died.

And these were but three of innumerable instances. The misery and need of people touched us wherever we moved when we lived overseas.

These last years we have lived in North America. Our home is attractive and comfortable. Clothes cram my closet. I struggle constantly against weight gain. Often I am deeply troubled wondering how I can call myself a Christian and have so much when others have so little.

Or I look out my study window and think of all my neighbors—dear people though they are!—whose lives give little evidence of faith in Jesus, and about the only thing I do about it is pray. Most of my time and energy are consumed in ministering to those who call themselves God's children and who have ample help already available to them. Is it right, I ask myself, to continue pouring all my energies into ministering to people who already know Christ? Shouldn't I be reaching out?

I sometimes wonder also what it really will be like to be ushered into the presence of God. If others "fell at his feet as though dead," will I do less? And if thoughts like this trouble me when I am well, at times of illness, when I am forced to face my mortality, God becomes "desperately real and shatteringly near" as the Hebrew scholar Abraham Herschel has noted concerning the prophets.

Have I ever had doubts about continuing life after death? Maybe it would be more accurate to say uncertainties and questions have arisen. Standing at the open coffin of my mother and looking at that still form, both so familiar and so unfamiliar, I was overwhelmed with a sense of the unknown. Where *was* mother? It was clear to me she wasn't in the coffin. But where was she then? In what form? The Bible is strangely silent on specific details.

I ventured to express these thoughts to some friends one day. One was silent and stared. Three exploded in surprise and shocked protest. One said quietly, "I can understand."

The three who had exploded immediately told me they were sure my mother was in heaven, safe and happy. One even suggested she was "tuning in on us just now."

I asked quietly on what part of Scripture they based this.

One recalled the verse, "Today you will be with me in paradise" (Luke 23:43). The one who had accepted my statement without judgment asked how this could be reconciled with the credal statement that Jesus "descended into hell"? Embarrassed laughter followed. My friend admitted that while this thought had occurred to her too, she guessed she hadn't wanted to struggle with it.

But then they proceeded to cite testimonies of those who had been near death who had claimed to have had visions of beautiful places and heavenly music. Mother herself had had an experience of this many years ago following surgery. She had recounted it often, and it had comforted her. But now my friends were basing their faith on experiences of others.

"Was this not risky?" I asked. Did we base any other of our Christian faith solely on human experience? Did we not base our faith primarily on what God had revealed in the Word? Did they find the question where my mother was now so threatening and unsettling that they couldn't struggle with it or even tolerate it?

"But why?" I asked. In the end we only *believe* in the resurrection of the dead and eternal life. We have no scientific proof, do we?

They talked then of Christ's own historical resurrection. "Ah, but you see," I said, "that isn't really what my problem is just now. I believe Christ is alive now—but I honestly don't know where mother is." It's the uncertainty of not knowing what happens to us immediately after death that was troubling me.

Another anxiety used to trouble me more some years ago than it does now, though I still think about it. When I hear statistics on average age expectancy, I catch myself counting how many years I can expect to have left. I begin to realize that I shall not be able to attain all that I have longed for. My most deeply cherished goals always elude me. I have attained lesser goals along the way, but am conscious of my imperfections and of how much more I could have done. The years seem to be slipping by so swiftly. I wonder if I have attained that for which Christ Jesus laid hold of me. Will I ever attain? There are so few years left!

How have I dealt with these troubling thoughts?

In the first place, I am not sure that I really can come to grips with my own death until it actually is imminent or unavoidable for me. Still I do think about it. Nor am I sure how I shall face it when that time comes. I do know that I shall have my God there beside me to help me through this difficult time.

It has helped me also to understand that, for Christians, death can carry a different meaning than it can for non-Christians. If we have been heeding Paul's injunction to die to ourselves but live to God, we have been in the process of dying and experiencing Christ's resurrection life for a long time. Death then becomes but the final event in a process that has been meant to go on a lifetime. As Thielicke said, death's threat is reduced to "the lower status of a background extra on the stage of life."

In my search for answers to my other anxieties I have turned to God, to God's Word, and to prayer. In regard to my anxieties about facing my judge and giving account, I turn to certain portions of Scripture and listen to them. Romans 8:1: "Therefore, there is now no condemnation for those who are in Christ Jesus, because through Christ Jesus the law of the Spirit of life set me free from the law of sin and death." Romans 6:23: "For the wages of sin is death, but the gift of God is eternal life in Christ Jesus our Lord." John 3:17-18: "For God did not send his Son into the world to condemn the world, but to save the world through him. Whoever believes in him is not condemned."

I know that when I appear before my judge, I shall have nothing of my own to cling to or present to him. But I will cling to the sacrificial death of him, who, though my judge, is also my Savior.

How do I deal with the feelings of overwhelming awe and fear that come as I think of one day standing in the presence of a holy, all-powerful, all-knowing God, infinitely greater than I can begin to imagine? For reassurance I turn to the Gospels. I see Jesus at work. I listen to him talk. I note his love, his concern, even his humor. And I know that if God is like his Son, I need not fear.

And what about my anxieties as to how far short my life falls in being like my Master has commanded? What about the abundance I enjoy? Again I turn to the Bible and I see Jesus not only caring for the poor, but feasting with the wealthy. I see Jesus celebrating at a wedding and providing more wine when some may have asked if the guests already had not had enough. I see Jesus accepting the extravagant gift of a woman. And I pray for grace both to enjoy the cup of plenty and to face the empty cup of need, even as I pray for willingness to share more and wisdom to know how to do it prudently.

Then there is the insecurity of not knowing what will happen to me after I leave my body. The evening after I had expressed my questionings as to where mother was after she had died, I turned once again to the verses mother had asked to be read at her funeral service. A verse from Ephesians 1 reads: "Having believed, you were marked in him with a seal, the promised Holy Spirit, who is a deposit guaranteeing our inheritance until the redemption of those who are God's possession—to the praise of his glory."

That word steadied me. I *know* I have received God's Spirit, for how else could I even believe in him? I know that I cannot by my own reason or strength even believe. Faith is a gift. But the fact that faith has taken up residence in my heart is my pledge, my assurance of a life beyond. What form that life will take immediately after death or even later I do not know for sure. But do I need to know that as long as I can trust a loving God?

Nor do I have to feel alarmed or unchristian if doubts come. Many of God's saints have experienced severe temptations as death has drawn near. Catherine of Siena was a mystic, prophet, and preacher in the 1300s. During the course of her life she became one of the most fearless, powerful, and effective preachers of her time. Thousands gathered to hear her. Hundreds were converted and scores healed. But her last days were agonizing. Her faith wavered as Satan, the Accuser, hurled accusation after accusation at her.

"I have sinned, Lord! Have mercy on me!" she cried out repeatedly.

Only at the very end did release come. Peace enveloped her. "Father, into your hands I commend my spirit," she cried. She was only 33 when she died.

And many other of God's people have confessed to times of doubting. Martin Luther admitted, "Sometimes I believe, and sometimes I doubt." Dostoevski confessed, "It is not as a child that I believe and confess Jesus Christ. My 'hosanna' is born in a furnace of doubt."

So if doubts assail me, I need not fear I have "lost faith." I can balance the comparatively few days and hours of wrestling with torturing doubts against all the days and weeks and months and years lived with a steady, trusting faith in God.

Henri Nouwen's words in his book *A Letter of Consolation* also have helped me through my struggle with vagrant feelings of revulsion and fear as I have thought of my own death. Nouwen notes that he came to understand why it is wrong to think that a death without struggle and agony is a sign of great faith. This idea, he declares, does not make much sense "once we realize that faith opens us to the full affirmation of life and gives us an intense desire to live more fully, more vibrantly, and more vigorously. If anyone should protest against death it is the religious person, the person who has increasingly come to know God as the God of the living."

So in regard to my concern that I shall not attain that for which "the Lord laid hold on me," I recognize that this may be an adventure that will never be fully consummated this side of death. The apostle Paul wrote, "I have finished the race, I have kept the faith" (2 Tim. 4:7). Keeping the faith is the important thing.

We should note also that not all experience anxiety as they consider death. When one has lived a long life and life no longer holds meaning or when living means suffering intense, hard-to-control pain, death can be welcomed and even prayed for. And even some who have not reached those stages are able to view death positively. The apostle Paul did. He wrote that he believed nothing could be better than to be with his Lord. Jeanne Crumley wrote that she was blessed with a sort of calm. "The possibility of death became very real to me," she said, "but in a comforting rather than a terrifying way."

As we walk up to or through the valley of the shadow of death, whether we enjoy this calming assurance or whether we are tortured with doubts and anxieties, we can cry out with the psalmist: "You are with me; your rod and your staff, they comfort me. . . . Surely goodness and love will follow me all the days of my life, and I will dwell in the house of the Lord forever" (Ps. 23:4, 6).

Helps for Your Quiet Times with the Lord

We acquaint ourselves with what the Lord says

Read Philippians 4:6. What is the antidote to anxiety given here?

Read Matthew 6:25-34. In this passage what does Jesus say we should do in order not to be anxious?

Read 1 Peter 5:7. What are we urged to do with our anxieties?

We reflect and meditate

One cannot sing "Gloria in Excelsis . . ." until one has first been helped to deal with one's fear.   ERNEST E. BRUDER

If I did not see that the Lord kept watch over the ship, I should long since have abandoned the helm. But I see Him! Through the storm He is strengthening the tackling, handling the yards, spreading the sails—aye more, commanding the very winds. Should *I* not be a coward if I abandoned *my* post? Let Him govern, let Him carry me forward, let Him hasten or delay. I will fear nothing!   MARTIN LUTHER

We pray

O most loving Father, you want us to give thanks for all things, to fear nothing except losing you and to lay all our cares on you, knowing that you care for us. Protect us from faithless fears and worldly anxieties, and grant that no clouds in this mortal life may hide from us the light of your immortal love shown to us in your Son, Jesus Christ our Lord. Amen.

Lutheran Book of Worship   prayer 204

The Significance
of the Silent Hours

In 1182 in the little walled Italian city-state Assisi, Lady Pica Bernadone, wife of Pierto, a wealthy cloth merchant, gave birth to a son, Francis.

Francis' boyhood dream was to become an illustrious knight. He joined a gang of boisterous youth, sons of counts and dukes. The youths would spur their horses up and down the narrow, winding, cobblestoned streets of Assisi. When the townsfolk heard them coming, they would flatten themselves against the walls of shops or flee in terror.

"Tell your son to be more careful," they pleaded with Pierto. But Pierto only laughed carelessly and said, "Boys will be boys," and did not rebuke his son. Francis' mother grieved and hoped for a better life for her son.

On the battlefield, when blood crimsoned the ground and the shrill screams of wounded men and whinnies of frightened horses chilled all who heard them, Francis' dream of fame and chivalry wavered. Later severe illness caused his dream to die completely. Francis' search for meaning in life began.

During his long convalescence he sat in the sun and reflected on his life. He noted that the only thing that really brought him satisfaction was talking with, listening to, and feeding the poor and the outcast who came to his gate. Wisely he paid attention to what he was finding to be deeply rewarding for him.

When he recovered sufficiently, he made a trip to Rome. There, too, he discovered it was not the impressive cathedrals but rather the poor at their gates that tugged at his heart. The assurance grew that he was moving in the right direction. He tested his heart leanings further. One day impulsively he exchanged clothes with a beggar. All day he sat in the beggar's place begging, trying to imagine what it would be like to be poor.

But he was to discover that that which attracted him repelled him also, that there was a limit to his natural compassion and that more than an attraction to the destitute would be needed. When he returned home, an encounter with a begging leper jarred him into this realization. As the disfigured leper approached him, Francis drew back in horror. Wheeling his horse around, he spurred away, pausing only long enough to throw back his purse to the leper still standing with fingerless hands outstretched.

But moments later he was stricken with remorse. The apostle Paul's words, "If I give all I possess to the poor . . . but have not love, I gain nothing," flashed into his mind, piercing and convicting him. He wheeled his horse around and galloped back to the beggar. Jumping off his horse, he knelt down and kissed the astonished beggar's hand. Relief, peace, and love flooded his being.

Convinced that he was acting in obedience to God, Francis

101

now took the final decisive steps. He told his father he wanted to give his life ministering to the poor. Horrified, his father locked him up. When his father left on a business trip, his mother set him free. Francis sought asylum at the bishop's house. When his father returned, Francis made public declaration of his intent in the town square, casting his clothes and the little money he had at his father's feet, declaring, "From now on I call God my Father."

Simple living, wholesome humor, lighthearted singing, caring for the poor and lepers, reconciling the estranged, bringing healing to the embittered, and living in close harmony with all nature characterized the remainder of Francis' life. Francis let the silent hours of his illness and recuperation determine the direction of his life. When he discovered that caring for the uncared for was the most important thing in life to him, he resolutely decided that would have priority regardless of the cost.

Gerald Strickler was in his teens when rheumatic fever gripped his body, forcing him to bed from May until September. "It was the year before sulfa and penicillin appeared on the market," he said. "I was glad I recovered."

But the illness left him with a damaged heart. Jerry had loved sports passionately and had dreamed of becoming a forest ranger. Now he had to abandon both of these interests. "But I was surprised how easy it was to relinquish them," he said. "Illness has a way of relaxing our hold on things."

He admits he experienced a sense of relief too at not having to enter military service. His damaged heart prevented that. Instead he was able to begin his college education. Even at that point he was able to see how good could come out of illness. Being able to enter college to train for the ministry compensated for having to abandon his dream of becoming a forest ranger. Actually, he confesses with a smile, becoming a minister perhaps was more in tune with God's will for him. He had felt nudgings in that direction earlier, and a number of people, recognizing his gifts, had encouraged him to enter the ministry. But until his illness he had resisted and tried to silence the call. During the long months in bed, with nothing to do but read and think, he had to face the call again. This time he acquiesced. Jerry's life was prolonged further when in his adult years he became one of the first persons in Southern California to have an aortic valve implant through surgery. But the rewarding ministry Jerry has had both as parish pastor and university professor of philosophy and religion has confirmed to him how right was the decision he made during the silent hours of his illness.

How much thought and prayer have we given to what is most important to us? Have we let God direct our choices? What are the driving forces in our lives?

If we have merely drifted into the work we are doing, if we have given preference to doing what has been expected of us by others, or what has been necessary to attain popularity, promotions, status, wealth, or security, we may have been conscious of vague feelings of discontent and dissatisfaction.

"I went home from my job every night and sat on my bed and cried," a young woman told me recently. "I thought the difficulties of my new job were getting me down. But as I became more honest with myself, I realized my deep unhappiness came as a result of the life I was living. When I decided to be through with a life that was in conflict with values I had learned in church during my childhood and youth—and which I was now realizing were the values I cherished most—peace flooded my heart."

Many of us, as we have moved along in life, have begun to turn a deaf ear to the voice of God speaking to us in the deepest recesses of our selves. As we have continued to do so, we have heard his voice less and less. The Holy Spirit, in turn, receiving such inhospitable treatment, has become more and more quiet. Busy schedules, ambitions, exciting vacations, and heavy responsibilities all can effectively silence him. Even a continuous round of church activities can block out God's voice. Christian workers too can become spiritually sterile and insensitive to the Holy Spirit.

Though we may not spend time consciously thinking about it, still the gap between what we are and what, way down deep, we know we would like to be, can produce subtle but destructive tension. Often we delay in probing for the real cause of the tension until illness results. Then the usual routine of life comes to a sudden halt. The noisy "silencers" to God's voice disappear. Laid aside, we can no longer be going, going, going or doing, doing, doing. We find ourselves having to live through many silent hours, forced to think. During this time the voice of God can again begin to assert itself. C. S. Lewis noted that God whispers to us in our pleasure, speaks to us in our conscience, but shouts in our pain.

What we learn during those quiet hours may vary greatly.

Many claim that the quiet hours of illness introduced themselves to their true selves.

"We do not know ourselves," Horatius Bonar stated. "Our convictions of sin have been but shallow, and we are beginning to think we have rid ourselves of many of our sins entirely, and are in a fair way speedily getting rid of all the rest. The depths of sin in us we have never sounded.

"Then the trial came. It swept over us like a cloud of the night, or rather through us like an icy blast, piercing and chilling us to our vitals. Then the old man within us awoke, and as if in response to the uproar without, a fierce tempest broke loose within. Unbelief arose in its former strength. Rebelliousness raged in every region of our soul. Unsubdued passions resumed their strength. We were dismayed at the fearful scene. Alas, we knew not the strength of sin nor the evil of our hearts till suddenly they broke loose."

Later he added, "The will is the seat of rebelliousness. At conversion the will is bent in the right direction, but it is still crooked and rigid. Rebelliousness is still there. Prosperous days may sometimes conceal it so that we are almost unconscious of its strength. But it still exists. Furnace heat is needed for softening and strengthening it."

Understanding the possibility of evil that lurks within each of us is basic to becoming authentic persons.

The temptation to worship gods other than the eternal Creator can come in subtle, sophisticated ways. Alan Redpath, pastor of a number of large congregations, experienced this when he was stricken with an almost fatal illness. After healing and restoration he wrote of the deep cleansing he had experienced. "The Lord showed me that I was putting work before worship," he said. "I had become much more concerned about the knowledge of truth than the knowledge of God."

Sometimes when we are ill, the Holy Spirit reminds us of sins with which we need to deal. Paul Lindell told of visiting a pastor who was very ill. He began to weep and confess a sin that had been eating away at him like acid. They talked together about God's merciful forgiveness.

"The peace of God fell upon him like a gentle rain," Paul said. "With great relief he sank back upon his pillows and said that now he was ready to die. But he didn't. God raised him up and gave him many more years of fruitful service."

"The purging of the soul is a mercy vouchsafed to a few . . . and to us who are sick falls the painful privilege of finding that our sufferings can become the flame which burns away the dross in our soul," wrote France Pastorelle.

"Earthly things and possessions meant less and less," another confessed, speaking of his time of illness. "Suddenly what mattered most was my life with Jesus."

If illness can help us release our hold on whatever has assumed God's place in our lives and if we reach out to grasp and hang on to the eternal, then surely we can thank God for illness.

Helps for Your Quiet Times with the Lord

We acquaint ourselves with what the Lord says

Read Psalm 51. What confession does David make? What requests does David make? What concept of God does David have?

We reflect and meditate

Sickness takes us aside and sets us alone with God and with all the props removed, we learn to lean on God alone. Often nothing but adversity will do this for us.   HORATIUS BONAR

In the majority of cases those who have gone through sorrow or suffering have received their "self" in its fires. That is not the same as saying that they have been made better by it. Sorrow and suffering do not necessarily make a person better; they burn up a great amount of shallowness; they give me myself or they destroy me.   OSWALD CHAMBERS

As light increases we see ourselves to be worse than we thought. . . . But we must neither be amazed nor disheartened.

We are not worse than we were; on the contrary, we are better.
. . . We only perceive our malady when the cure begins.

FRANCOIS FENELON

We pray

Use Psalm 51 as your prayer. Follow it with your own prayer of thanksgiving for the forgiveness God offers us in Jesus.

Integrating Illness into Our Lives

In a great music hall in Germany the wild applause of the audience drowned out the last notes of Beethoven's Ninth Symphony. But the conductor stood, still facing his orchestra, head bowed, baton lowered. Finally an orchestra member stepped forward. Taking his conductor by the arm, he turned him around so he could see the hats and handkerchiefs being waved and the ecstatic joy on the faces of the people.

The conductor was Ludwig von Beethoven. The melody that had evoked such tumultuous response was the one to which we now sing, "Joyful, joyful we adore you!"

Beethoven himself had heard it only in the imagination of his mind. He had tried, through music, to interpret his long and anguished journey in integrating his tragic affliction of deafness into the fabric of his life. The way had been stormy and painful, full of angry outbursts, laments, and complaints. But he had persisted, and so thoroughly had he completed his task that he could end on a note of ecstatic joy.

When he first had become aware of his hearing disability

in 1798, he had written to a friend, "Your Beethoven is most unhappy and at strife with nature and the Creator."

For some time Beethoven had refused to accept the seriousness of his increasing impairment. But as his hearing had declined, he finally had been forced to face his problem. He had begun to withdraw socially, for, he had said, "It is impossible for me to say to people, 'I am deaf.'" Because he did not tell people about his disability, he had found people lacking in understanding. They thought he had become absent-minded. In reality he simply had not heard what they had said.

People's attitudes began to annoy, then provoke him to anger. Anger drove him to determine to overcome his disability by stubborn, though unreasonable, self-determination. "I will take Fate by the throat," he shouted. But Beethoven was up against something he could not conquer.

Although he wondered how he could ever compose music again, he still felt there was more for him to do. Nor could he believe that he could be happy again if he could not compose music.

"O Providence," he wrote in his journal, "grant me at last one day of pure joy—it is so long since real joy echoed in my heart—Oh, when—Oh, when, O Divine One, shall I find it again in the temple of nature and of men? Never? No—Oh, that would be too hard!"

Nevertheless, he began to recognize that his illness was compelling him to become what otherwise he perhaps would not have become, at least not to as great a degree. "Forced already in my 28th year to become a philosopher," he wrote.

That enforced reflection on life, illness, pain, and suffering was to bring to his music a richness, an honesty, and an integrity it could not have had otherwise. But growth in integrating illness, pain, and suffering into his life came step by step even after he began consciously to assimilate it into his life. Slowly he moved from finding meaning in life *in spite of* suffering to finding the deepest meaning in life *in* suffering. He saw illness not as an intrusion, but recognized the possibility of integrating it into his life, thereby transforming something basically evil into something good.

If illness is to play a meaningful role for us, our task will be to integrate it into the fabric of our lives. How we integrate it, the difficulty or ease with which we integrate it, and the extent of its influence on our lives is determined by a number of different factors: our backgrounds, ages, intelligence, emotional development, religious beliefs, personalities, and past experiences with illness, suffering, death, or adversity.

"I was blessed because I never felt the need to know *why* I had cancer," Jeanne Crumley said. "I did not feel I had to pin the blame on myself or God or Satan or others. I was enabled by God, I think, to accept what happened and to use my energy not in questioning it but in dealing with it."

Jeanne is young and intelligent. She grew up in a godly home. During her illness she said she could not pinpoint any particular time when she felt especially close to God, but throughout she was conscious of his presence and help and believed her illness had drawn her closer to him.

Physiological problems will affect whether or not we are able to integrate illness into our lives. Brain damage, for example, distorts judgment. We may think we are able to carry on our work when we are not. We may imagine that we are not ill when we are. Needless to say, those in that condition will not be giving much thought to finding meaning in an illness which they are convinced they do not have.

Excessive weakness can also prevent one from searching for meaning in what is happening.

"I was so weak," one cancer patient said, "that I couldn't even listen to music or think or even wonder why I was sick. I just sat or lay."

For some, integrating illness into one's life is almost an unconscious absorption of it, possible because of unquestioning acceptance of it. For others, it results only after a mighty, tumultuous, stormy, fist-shaking, finger-waving, name-calling battle. Wearied and worn, the combatants finally lay down their swords and are ready to surrender. At that point, if they are able, not simply to resign themselves to what has happened, but to accept it, they take the first important step in integrating their illness into their lives.

Dr. Paul Tournier points out that "Resignation is passive. Acceptance is active. Resignation abandons the struggle against suffering. Acceptance strives but without rebellion. . . . Still there is no attitude more impossible for people— without the miraculous intervention of Christ—than the acceptance of suffering of any kind."

Without acceptance, however, integration will be impossible.

The second thing necessary, if illness is to be integrated into our lives, is reflection. Many remain impoverished and gain nothing from difficult times because they refuse to reflect.

"I don't want to talk about it. It's past," they say. "I want to forget all about it."

Samuel Rutherford protested that we should not do so. "Truly no cross should be old to us," he wrote. "We should not forget them because years are come betwixt us and our crosses. We should not cast them away as we do old clothes. We may make a cross old in time, new in use and as fruitful as in the beginning of it."

Horatius Bonar agreed. "We look on trials too much as we

do upon a passing shower which falls and then is gone," he wrote. "The benefits of chastisement should never be exhausted. Even when sitting calmly in the sunshine we may be drawing profit from the stormy past."

Indeed, often it is only after we are far removed from the time of suffering that we can perceive the good that has come. To begin with, the memories of pain-wracked nights, of hideous nausea, and of frightening weakness are too vivid. They fill the mind and memory's screen. And if the illness has robbed us of mobility, agility, speech, sight, limbs, or beauty, we shall need to utilize time at first to mourn our loss. Our bloodless wounds are too fresh for us to give attention to anything else.

But after a while wounds close over and heal. Pain eases. Anxieties lessen. Questions may remain, but they no longer are shouting for answers. Then it is that we can begin to review and reflect. And reflect we must if we are going to draw sweet waters from our well of pain.

Another factor in our ability to integrate illness into our lives is our environment. Our environment can either assist or hinder us in our search for meaning. Is it one that gives us a feeling of security and makes it possible for us to rest and reflect? Am I surrounded by those who love me, and do they take my illness in stride so that I do not feel I am burdening them? Am I facing more than one crisis so my energy is depleted and my attention distracted?

Time is needed for integration. Sometimes we need a lifetime in order to perceive the full effect integration of our illness has had on our entire life. Pastor Edwin Petrusson, now in his late 70s, can trace how illness shaped his whole life.

In early manhood, just as he was approaching the end of his training for the ministry, he came down with tuberculosis.

He had never experienced disappointment before, he said, but the 17 months he lay ill became a time of wonderful preparation for the ministry.

During the long hours when there was not much else to do than think, he came to understand what it means to lose everything one has taken for granted: health, strength, future plans. He was engaged to be married. Now even marriage seemed problematic.

However, young though he was, he realized that sooner or later most people come to terms with the fragility of life and that his experience was not exceptional.

To help the time pass, he enrolled in Bible correspondence courses that emphasized Scripture memorization. He learned hundreds of Bible verses, and often would lie and meditate on them. "It gave me a rich treasury," he said, "but one not only for my own enrichment. Later in preaching I could quote readily by heart."

The correspondence courses also taught him the value of teaching. After recovery, teaching became a central focus of his parish ministry. Later his interest in teaching led to full-time teaching in a Bible institute for 22 years.

One of the correspondence courses was in personal witnessing. Taking the course encouraged him to witness freely and enabled him to do so. "And again all the Scripture memorizing I had done proved helpful," he said.

"Because I myself had been ill so long, later, after recovery, I felt at home in hospitals," he added. "This also helped me in my parish work."

Thus, in retrospect, Pastor Petrusson has been able to see how his illness has affected his whole lifetime. The fruitful ministry he has enjoyed came, not in spite of illness, but because of it.

I too can trace the effect illness and the death of a sister, father, mother, my dearest friend, and two sons have had on my ministry. Because of these experiences I can feel comfortable with those who are suffering. I am at home in a hospital or at the bedside of someone dying. And though I have not consciously planned it thus, as I review my writings, I can see how many of them have dealt with illness, pain, death, and bereavement.

But I believe illness also has had less visible but more profound effects on my life, bringing about changes in my person. Life in the past sometimes was bumpy and stormy for me because I was both strong-willed and self-willed, easily angered and frustrated when things did not go my way. That has changed. I *want* God's will now and am willing to accept what he sends without insisting that I have to understand all the "whys" and "wherefores." Being the stubborn, untamed creature I was, I believe that only some hard knocks could domesticate me to the point where I was willing to bow my head and let the Lord slip his yoke over my head so it would rest on my shoulders. It feels good there now.

Illness and bereavement have changed my relationship to God. I think of my posture before God now most often to be one of worship. In one sense there is a greater distance between God and me than before. It is right and proper that there be this distance. He is God. I am just a very tiny Christian and just one of millions of Christians. I am awed and humbled that, considering all who have never heard of him, I should be one granted that privilege. And knowing how many struggle to believe, I also am grateful for faith. So I rejoice to be one of God's dearly loved children, but I also realize I am only one and that God loves all—and even those outside the fold—as much as he loves me.

God's ways are more mysterious for me than ever, but what

I cannot understand now causes me to wonder and marvel more than to doubt.

I think that adversity does not upset me as much as formerly, but I am not sure about this. Life just now is pleasant. If tragedy struck, how would I react? I can only trust God to see me through.

Life itself surely has become one of my most highly prized treasures. I greet every morning with joy and anticipation—after a shower has awakened me! I am strongly motivated to work because I am conscious how fragile and uncertain life is and that I have no guarantee as to how much remaining time I might have.

I deeply value and cherish my family. They always have had priority in my life and will continue to occupy a prominent place. Perhaps the very difficulty with which our family circle was formed has made me cherish it so deeply. The home I grew up in enriched me. As I grew to young adulthood, more than anything else I wanted a home, a husband, and children. I had to wait until I was 30 before I met my husband. Only through much difficulty, anxiety, pain, and sorrow did we get our four children.

Also I believe, through my various illnesses which have occasioned serious reflection, a good bit of my ego-centered ambition has disappeared. I still want to write, communicate, and influence; perhaps the desire is stronger than ever. But I think I have been set free, at least to a significant degree, from distracting, enervating absorption with measuring my "success" or worth against published records of best-sellers. I know that I must write what is authentically mine. I must write what I believe regardless of how well it will be accepted or how widely it will sell. Slowly I think I am learning also to accept that I do not need to write like someone else. I may and do admire the styles of other writers, but again I must be true to myself and my style—simple though it may be.

I think that my illnesses also have helped me to be more open to learning. Differing opinions do not threaten me as much any more, so I can read more widely and listen to those with whom I differ. Along with that I do not arrogantly believe that I and only I have the right answers or that only I perceive things correctly. But I have to believe enough in what I do believe so that I will not hesitate to state my convictions.

Integration of illness into one's life, I recognize also, may be spasmodic and transitory. The lessons I think I have learned I may have to relearn. Beethoven struggled with maintaining an attitude of constantly and consistently accepting his disability and integrating it at all times into his life.

As we reflect and seek to be taught by God, we may notice other subtle changes taking place within us also. We find strange, new tender feelings toward others filling our hearts. We eagerly seek out others who are hurting. Sickness, pain, suffering, and even death no longer frighten us. We feel comfortable and at home with people who are suffering. We discover also that we are apologizing for people more frequently than we are criticizing them. What has happened? When we were not looking, tolerance, compassion, and patience have stolen into our hearts and taken up residence there.

None of us likes illness or suffering. But both are an inescapable part of life. Katherine Mansfield, writing in her journal, declared: "I should like this to be accepted as my confession. There is no limit to human suffering. When one thinks: 'Now I have touched the bottom of the sea—now I can go no deeper,' one goes deeper. . . . But I do not want to die without leaving a record of my belief that suffering can be overcome. For I do believe it. What must one do? One must submit. Do not resist. Take it. Be overwhelmed. Accept it fully. Make it part of life."

Helps for Your Quiet Times with the Lord

We acquaint ourselves with what the Lord says

Read Romans 8:28. Memorize this wondrous promise.

We reflect and meditate

I saw a cup sent down and come to her
    Brimful of loathing and of bitterness;
She drank with livid lips that seemed to stir
    The depth, not make it less.
But as she drank I spied a Hand distill
    New wine and virgin honey; making it
First bitter-sweet, then sweet indeed, until
    She tasted only sweet.
    CHRISTINA ROSSETTI

We pray

Almighty God, to whom our needs are known before we ask: Help us to ask only what accords with your will; and those good things which we dare not or, in our blindness, cannot ask, grant us for the sake of your Son, Jesus Christ our Lord. Amen.
    Lutheran Book of Worship   prayer 211

Harvesting Our Illness

Out of illness we can reap a rich harvest. Life itself becomes inexpressibly precious when we have been threatened with having it end for us. However, not only life itself, but all the little pleasures of life, which we had taken for granted before, become objects of profound gratitude.

"Several weeks after surgery I announced one afternoon that I was hungry for a bacon, lettuce, and tomato sandwich," Ione Johnson wrote. "Herb went to the store. When I had it all ready, I looked at that beautiful sandwich, thanked the Lord, and cried. That was the best meal I've had in my entire life."

One's sensory perceptions are heightened also. Dr. Hans Zinsser was a biologist known chiefly for his isolation of the germ of typhus. He himself contracted an incurable disease of the blood and knew for over a year that he was dying. In his autobiography *As I Remember Him,* written in the third person, he tells of standing with a friend looking out at the Charles River Basin in Lowell, Massachusetts. It was a June day, early afternoon. Bright sunshine was reflected on the water. Sailboats skimmed by. On the shores people strolled. The laughter of children floated through the windows to the place where the two friends stood. In those few minutes, Dr. Zinsser said, a change took place within him.

In the prospect of death, life seemed to be given new meaning and fresh poignancy. It seemed, he said, "that from that moment, as though all that his heart felt and his senses perceived were taking on a deep autumnal tone and an increased vividness. From now on, instead of being saddened, he found, to his own delighted astonishment, that his sensitivity to the simplest experiences, even for things that in other years he might hardly have noticed, was infinitely enhanced. When he awoke in the mornings, the early sun striking across the bed, the noise of the sparrows, and all the sounds of the awakening street aroused in him all kinds of gentle and pleasing memories of days long past which had left their imprints of contentment and happiness. He felt a deeper tenderness for the people whom he loved, and a warmer sympathy and understanding for many whose friendship he had lost in one way or another. Each moment of the day, every prospect on meadow or hill or sea, every change of light from dawn to dusk, excited him emotionally with an unexpected clarity of perception and a new suggestiveness of association. Everything that went on about him or within him struck upon his heart and mind with a new and powerful resonance."

The forced inactivity of illness also may lead to a new appreciation as to what makes a person worthwhile.

"I learned that my worth as a person is not attributed so much to my daily activities or what I am able to *do,* but rather what I *am,* the attitudes and opinions and values that make up my personality," Jeanne Crumley wrote.

119

Illness can teach us how dependent we are on God and others. We become more human.

"I have become aware of my own limitations to a greater degree. I no longer feel the need to deny them. Instead I can find ways to work through them creatively," Jeanne Crumley said. And then she added, "I feel I grew spiritually during my illness also. I was forced to acknowledge my dependence on Someone greater than myself. I was challenged by something which alone I could not conquer. It's been a subtle thing; it was not revolutionary or even readily apparent to others, but it has changed me."

Clara Carlson shared the same thoughts. "Through my illness I learned how much we are dependent upon one another. We may pride ourselves on being independent, but life is not like that. Life becomes a sharing and caring experience. We never walk alone. I also learned trustful living—trust not in my own self, but in Christ who loves and cares for me far above what I can ever ask, think, or imagine."

Countless great men and women in history, who suffered ill health throughout much of their lives and yet achieved, discovered that indeed we are made strong in weakness. Theodore Fliedner, father of the deaconess movement, survived typhoid fever and smallpox attacks and spent months, at various times, in tuberculosis sanatoriums. Finally, life-long bronchial infection caused him to spend his last months in the humid ammonia atmosphere of a cow barn where breathing seemed easier. When he finally died at age 64, his ventures had grown into 22 institutions at his center in Kaiserwerth, Germany. The 425 deaconesses he had trained at the Kaiserwerth Motherhouse were busily at work—including Florence Nightingale. Seventy-five years later the Kaiserwerth General Conference listed 35,000 deaconesses. In addition, at that time 10,000 in the Protestant churches traced their beginnings to the Kaiserwerth Motherhouse. All of this from a man who repeatedly suffered ill health!

George Handel was recovering from a stroke and was still impaired by some paralysis when he wrote the *Messiah*, complete with the "Hallelujah Chorus." Creativity can be born out of despair.

Often at a time of illness one becomes aware of all the friends one has. "A friend asked one day if she could count all the cards I had received," Ione Johnson said. "There were over 500!"

Relationships can grow deeper through an experience of illness, though sometimes the route is through stormy waters.

Marge Wold, writing in *Thanks for the Mountain*, tells of the strain placed on her husband's and her relationship during the long period of recuperation following Erling's surfing accident in which he broke his neck. "The strain on our relationship was so intense at times that, except for the love we share, and the forgiveness the Spirit enables us to mutually give and receive, we could never have successfully kept that blithe pledge we had made so long ago before God's marriage altar."

At the same time illness often awakens feelings of deep tenderness toward everybody, even the unlovely.

"I hope my experience in my illness will continue to influence my sensitivity to others as I encounter them daily and enable me to be supportive and encouraging," Jeanne Crumley said.

Her father added: "Illness makes one more sensitive to the pain others bear. We become better ministers ourselves as we are ministered to. Illness is a time when other people can be invited into our lives, a time that prepares us to accept what others offer as it is offered, not just on our terms."

"The saint's willingness to suffer liberates the capacity for love," Caryll Houselander stated.

Illness can afford us opportunities to develop talents that have laid latent. Kagawa, the esteemed Japanese Christian who poured out his life for the poor, wrote a novel while he was recuperating from tuberculosis. So poor he couldn't afford paper, he brushed out his story over the pages of a magazine. But when it finally was published, it sold a quarter million copies and launched him as a writer.

Witnessing to one's faith often seems to come easier and more naturally when one is ill. A Korean friend, who had her entire stomach removed because of cancer, remarked several years later: "I lost just my stomach, but I gained so much! Because I suffered then, now when I visit others I can hold their hand, and they can hear me because I've been where they are. Even those who aren't suffering seem able to hear. The surgeon who performed my operation came to faith in Christ, and there have been others too."

"It would seem," another wrote, "that occasionally God allows illness for the benefit of others. To the atheist or agnostic, one of the best demonstrations of God is to see a child of his under stress. The difference in the life of the believer shows up best under pressure."

After we ourselves have been ill, the sickness and suffering of others no longer causes us to shrink back. "I began to cultivate the ability to approach suffering directly in a helpful, supportive way, rather than avoiding and downplaying it," Jeanne Crumley said.

"Sickness caused us to reach out to others in a practical way," one whose spouse had been seriously ill for a year said. "Now, even though our income has dropped sharply, we find both time and money to bake goods and prepare casseroles and go and visit the sick and their families. It has become one of our highest priorities."

Special diets, regular exercise, and rest which the doctor often prescribes teach us discipline and can help us establish better health habits.

Martin Luther claimed that "were it not for tribulation I could not understand Scripture." Experience does give insight into the Scriptures. Bible scholars say, for example, that Revelation was written for Christians under persecution. Evidently they understood it well, but for us in an affluent, comfortable situation it is often read but seldom understood. Maybe a little suffering would give us a better understanding of the last book of the Bible.

Strangely enough, illness also can make us profoundly grateful. Martin Rinkhart wrote the hymn "Now Thank We All Our God" in the midst of suffering. Much of his life was lived during the Thirty Years' War in the walled city of Eilenburg. People from all the country around sought refuge in the city. Overcrowding caused famine and pestilence. Rinkhart sometimes buried 40 or 50 persons in a day. His wife died, and he himself fell ill but survived. But out of that experience, incredible as it seems, came this magnificent hymn of praise.

Karolina Sandell wrote "Children of the Heavenly Father" in her teens while she was struggling to become mobile following an illness which had left her paralyzed.

Ludwig Helmbold wrote "From God Can Nothing Move Me" in the midst of a pestilence in Erfurt, Germany, that killed 4000. The hymn declares that "a troubled world rejoices each time we worship" God.

On the lighter side, a physician said that during his illness he learned to laugh at the clock. " 'Clock,' I would say in mock disdain, 'I don't have to pay any attention to you today.'

And for a busy physician that is a priceless luxury, even at the cost of one's health for a period of time."

Some are motivated to offer themselves as subjects for medical experimentation or research. A word of warning and caution is in order, however. Such research may place oneself and one's family under terrible stress. All need to understand completely what is involved.

Perhaps most of us miss discovering wherein the real spiritual struggle lies when we become ill. Russian Orthodox priest Dmitri Dudko declared, "In our earthly life a battle rages. The devil fights against God. The field of battle is man's heart, as Dostoevski said. The Christian isn't called a warrior for nothing."

If we understood and accepted the reality of the spiritual warfare going on when one who is God's child is being tested, we could get a better perspective on our suffering.

When we are ill our bodies may shrivel, but our souls can grow. We may be denied most of the things that the world prizes most highly, but the truly priceless and lasting things of life can unfold to us. Whatever we lose, if we gain wisdom, then we profit from our loss. The harvest we can reap from our illness is full-sheaved indeed.

Helps for Your Quiet Times with the Lord

We acquaint ourselves with what the Lord says

Read 1 Peter 1:6-9; 2 Corinthians 12:7-10; Psalm 103.

We reflect and meditate

It is misleading to imagine that we are developed in spite of our circumstances. We are developed because of them. It is mastery *in* circumstances that is needed, not mastery over them.

OSWALD CHAMBERS

One's philosophy is not best expressed in words; it is expressed in the choices one makes. . . . In the long run we shape our lives, and we shape ourselves. The process never ends until we die. And the choices we make are ultimately our responsibility. ELEANOR ROOSEVELT

We pray

What have you gained during your time of illness? Thank God for this.

They Tell Me It Could Have Been a Lot Worse

With a sigh and a groan the old Nepali man rested his heavily-laden bamboo basket on a high ledge under the spreading banyan tree. He slid the flat woven bamboo strap off his forehead and wiped away the perspiration with the back of his tattered sleeve. Then he lowered himself to a squatting position on the ground, still grasping his sturdy walking stick. Only then did he seem to notice me, sitting on the ground, resting my back against the ledge. His brown eyes surveyed me frankly.

We exchanged customary greetings. He had come to India to buy his family's yearly supply of salt, he said. Home was back in the mountains of Nepal, he said, pointing with his chin, three days' walking distance. He shifted his position. I was the first "pink-faced queen" he had ever seen or talked to, he confided. He had only heard of us before.

"Tell me," he said, "are you the same color here," pointing to his abdomen, "as you are here?" pointing to his face.

126

I obligingly pulled apart the blouse and skirt I was wearing to show him that I was indeed the same color all over.

Satisfied, he leaned back against the ledge. "Pink-faced queen," he said, "I have some questions to ask you."

Back in his country, he explained, he had neighbors who as Gurkha soldiers had served in other countries. They had returned from their ventures overseas with strange tales. He wanted to know if what they had told him was true. And so he asked me about the shape of the earth, about trains and submarines. And then he asked, "Pink-faced queen, I have heard there are very wise people in your country. They have power to cast people who are in pain into deep sleep. Then while the people sleep these wise ones cut open the spot where the pain is, remove the devil, sew up the opening, wake up the person, and the person is well. Is it so, Pink-faced queen?"

I smiled. "Yes, it is so, Grandfather, only let me explain it a bit more," I said.

He listened, stroking his beard as he listened, his brown eyes wide and thoughtful. In the end I asked him, "And how is it for you, Grandfather? When you are sick, what do you do?"

He shook his head sadly. "We?" he asked. "We have no one to give us understanding. We shake like leaves of the poplar tree in the wind when we get sick. We wonder who has cast a curse on us. We go to our village sorcerer and bring him chickens and rice and ask him to work magic to deliver us. And we chop the heads off some chickens and offer to the gods. And if we live, we live. If we die," his voice trailed off. He sat silent for a while, then touched the huge goiter on the side of his neck. "Could your wise men take care of this problem of mine?" he asked.

"Ah, yes," I said.

"That would be so good," he said, "so good."

127

I also remember a sick old lady who lived in India as well. She had been abandoned by her family and left alone to die because they were convinced evil spirits had taken possession of her. The first day I visited her she crouched in a corner of her dark hut.

"Don't you see them?" she asked, covering her face with her hands and crouching even lower. "They dance all around me, sneering and laughing, because they know they soon will get me."

We tried to declare to her God's liberating word. She listened and seemed to reach out briefly but then resumed her rocking and weeping.

"It's too late for me," she said. "Maybe if you had come earlier, it could have been different, but there is no hope for me."

For these two suffering sick ones—and there are thousands like them—sickness is a grievous burden.

And there was an age when illness could be considered only a burden, a punishment, or a curse. People were confused about what caused illness. They thought sickness meant a person had sinned or become possessed by evil spirits, and so they shrank from and abhorred the sick.

We find reference to this belief in the book of Job, which is believed to record some of our most ancient history. Job's friends were sure he would not be suffering if he had not sinned against God and broken his relationship with him.

"Those who sow trouble reap it," Eliphaz declared confidently. "At the breath of God they are destroyed" (Job 4:8-9).

Bildad suggested it was the sins of Job's sons that had brought about their accidental deaths.

"Does God pervert justice?" he asked. "Does the Almighty pervert what is right? When your children sinned against him, he gave them over to the penalty of their sin" (Job 8:3-4).

This attitude towards sickness was passed on from generation to generation. It was still common in Jesus' time as we see by a question Jesus' followers asked him. "Who sinned?" they asked, "this man or his parents, that he was born blind?" (John 9:2).

"Neither this man nor his parents sinned," said Jesus, but this happened so that the work of God might be displayed in his life" (John 9:3).

Jesus sought to correct people's understanding of and attitudes toward sickness. He taught, not only by verbal explanations, but also by the way he acted toward the suffering sick. He touched them, loved them, talked with them, and ministered to their deepest psychological and spiritual needs.

Jesus' approach to the sick left people talking and arguing. They were astonished, dumbfounded, amazed, and filled with questions. Some were upset because the old traditions and teachings were being questioned. Some, who were chronically ill, appear to have become so hardened from being scorned by people because they were ill that they did not know how to be grateful when Jesus healed them.

But, generally speaking, those who were sick or who had loved ones who were sick felt their hearts surge with joy and hope. Jesus' behavior toward the sick freed their legs to run to him. Here was one who accepted them, who did not push them off into a corner, who did not always blame their illness on evil powers. Here was one who healed and restored. His attitude, his concern, and his power left people wide-eyed.

A new attitude was brought to birth in the hearts of people. Instead of detesting the sick, Christ's followers began to love them. Instead of carrying them out to the forest to die, they began to care for them. Instead of abandoning them, they began to help them recover. Instead of berating and condemning them, they began to pray for them. Christ's bearing of our sicknesses removed from the suffering sick the heavy burden of being ostracized, criticized, condemned, shunned, abandoned, and abhorred. Through the centuries that follow we see that burden being lifted more and more in country after country as Jesus' teachings and the healing ministry of his followers change people's attitudes.

Even in our country people often are confused. When they become ill, many immediately wonder what sin they have committed to have this happen to them. Or if a loved one becomes ill, they wonder if they are responsible for that illness because of some sin of which they are guilty.

It is true that we may suffer from some illnesses because we have misused our bodies or minds. We also may suffer because others have misused or mistreated us. But generally speaking we suffer from illness simply because we are part of the human family, subject to the illnesses that came upon all mankind when Adam and Eve chose to go their own way rather than God's. So we may be assured that most of the time when we become ill or when a loved one becomes ill it is *not* because we have committed some particular sin.

Even though most people believe and accept this, yet unconsciously people may draw back from those who are ill. Toyohiko Kagawa, the compassionate advocate of the poor in Japan, wrote of his experience when the doctor discovered he had tuberculosis. "I had to retreat to a fishing village where I lived in a miserable cottage," he said. "Japanese didn't dare approach me."

In our country victims of disfiguring diseases, mentally ill people, and the elderly whose bodies have deteriorated—and sometimes even cancer victims—still feel shunned. A woman fighting cancer told of being served her punch in a paper cup at a party while others were served theirs in glasses! Change is coming, but slowly.

Our abhorrence of illness, kept carefully hidden most of the time, sometimes becomes visible in subtle ways, however. We hug a well person impulsively and warmly, and give them lingering kisses. When that person becomes sick, the hug becomes a pat, the kiss a quick exchange, then a peck. Gradually the peck is transferred from mouth to cheek to forehead and then finally blown from the tips of the fingers. So even for us, in many overt and covert ways, some of the stigma of being sick remains. The burden has not been lifted entirely.

But to a large extent the burden of being ostracized and despised when we are sick *has* been lifted from us. Kagawa experienced the burden being lifted when a Christian missionary doctor came to him. Kagawa wrote, "Dr. Myers came to me and slept with me on the floor four nights. I asked him whether he was not scared of tuberculosis. He said, 'No!' Dr. Myers knew I was lonesome. It was summer and terribly hot. We had many mosquitoes. His wife and children were in a summer resort far away, but leaving them, he came down to me in that burning hot place."

We today see the burden lifted from us by the hospitals, doctors, nurses, and medical staff of an astonishing variety who possess awesome skills and knowledge and now stand ready to care for us when we are ill. Chaplains, pastors, social workers, friends, and family members also care. Our employers provide plans to alleviate our financial needs when we are ill. We are surrounded by love, care, and healing skills. And we are supported.

In yet another aspect the burden of sickness has been lifted from us to an astonishing degree. We are a much healthier people than we were even a few years ago. Not as many of us get sick, we are not sick as often or as seriously ill as we were even 50 years ago, and we make faster and more complete recoveries.

Chances for survival in critical cases have improved immensely, and new ways of treatment have eliminated the need for some surgical procedures that formerly were psychologically traumatic.

Almost all of these strides towards wholeness have come as a result of Christ's coming, his teaching, and his compassionate attitude toward the sick. And what Jesus did, he did because he was in life-giving touch with the Father. "Whatever the Father does, the Son also does," he said (John 5:19). Loving and caring have been eternal concerns of the Father.

Later Jesus added, "Anyone who has faith in me will do what I have been doing. He will do even greater things than these, because I am going to the Father." Thus he made us partners with him in his healing ministry, though in one sense all healing still proceeds from him alone. Even doctors acknowledge this.

We need to remember also that any healing which we experience comes to us only at great cost. Our healing cost Christ more than we ever can imagine. "Surely he took up our infirmities [pains], and carried our sorrows [sickness]," we read in Isaiah 53. Do we not catch a little of his anguish at having to carry this burden in his cry, "My Father, if it is not possible for this cup to be taken away unless I drink it, may your will be done" (Matt. 26:42)? Healing comes to us only at great cost to Jesus Christ. "But he was pierced for our transgressions, he was crushed for our iniquities, the punishment that brought us peace was upon him, and by his wounds we are healed" (Isa. 53:5).

It is easier for us to understand that our healing has cost others something. Think of the long, exhausting hours doctors and other health professionals put in during their training. Think of the cost in terms of fatigue when emergencies arise and doctors are awakened after only a few hours sleep and summoned to perform several hours of surgery. Think of the cost in terms of mental, physical, and emotional strain to deal daily with life and death situations, the strain placed on family relationships.

"Doctors shouldn't marry," a surgeon said to me. "Our profession demands so much of us we have too little left to give of ourselves and our time to have good marriages." He knew. Twice his own marriage had ended in divorce. Doctors may be reimbursed generously for their work, but can money ever compensate for some of the price they pay?

Others have paid a price too. Think of the hours scientists have spent in lonely laboratories, experiencing frustration after frustration as they have tried to track down the cause of a disease. Think of the years spent developing vaccines and serums. Think of the lives laid down by those who offered their bodies for medical research. For example, yellow fever, to a large extent, has been brought under control. But before an effective vaccine finally was developed, the Rockefeller Foundation had spent more than 12 million dollars, and countless volunteers and at least half a dozen brilliant scientists had died.

So good health and healing come to us today only at inestimable cost, first to Christ and then to others. Too long have we talked only about how much it costs *us* to be sick.

Life for you and me when we are ill is much easier because of Jesus' teachings, his actions, and his bearing of our sicknesses on the cross. A changed attitude on the part of people has resulted. We in the Western world have not known the burden of being ostracized and abhorred when we become ill. To most of us it has not even occurred that we should not be loved, cared for, and helped to recover when we are ill. We have enjoyed this manifestation of the grace of God so long we have not even recognized it as grace. But it has come to us only at great cost, to Christ and others. We realize, in a new way, how much we are indebted to others, and we give thanks.

Helps for Your Quiet Times with the Lord

We acquaint ourselves with what the Lord says

Read Isaiah 41:10, 13; Psalm 103:8-18.

We reflect and meditate

In the world of the first-century Christians, the good are likely to suffer more, not less, in this life. The world is so topsy-turvy that suffering, far from being a result of sin, almost becomes the sign you are one of the faithful. . . . The majority of the New Testament texts . . . have given up on meanings in this world and have postponed the coming of God's justice until the time when Jesus comes again or we die.   DANIEL J. SIMUNDSON

(Ponder how we can relate this observation to what Christians in needy Third World countries and Christians in repressive countries today experience.)

Blessed are those who use their sorrow [illness] creatively, for they shall find a security that is not shaken by circumstances, but rather produces the fruits of enriched sympathy, heightened understanding and deepened faith.   EDGAR N. JACKSON

We pray

Spend a few moments thinking back to what it was like when your grandparents became ill. Thank God for all the progress that has been made and all the blessings that are yours now when you are ill. Take time to think one by one of all the good things going for you. How many can you name? Give thanks.

See Him! See Him!

We rejoice that healing continues to take place even though Christ is not a visible presence with us now. The fact that healing continues is a sign that God has not abandoned us. God continues active among us.

So see your Healer now. See Jesus at work.

He spends little time philosophizing about the origin of evil and suffering. Rather he sees people's need. He responds. He heals. He heals *people*. He doesn't see his chief object to be circumstantial conditions that need to be corrected. He doesn't talk about all the disease-carrying flies in Nazareth, the waters of Jericho polluted with human refuse, the malnutrition of hundreds. Not that this is to be ignored by us, but Jesus never became so engrossed in treating causes that he forgot the people involved. He never became more concerned about causes than people. Jesus' primary focus always was on people.

Read through the Gospels and notice how often it is noted that Jesus *saw* the sick. When he saw them, he stopped. The sick caught his attention. But he not only stopped. He asked, "What do you want me to do for you?" (Matt. 20:32). And when those he addressed responded that they wanted to be made well, Jesus had compassion on them. The word *compassion* is a strong one, meaning "feeling all chewed up inside." The sickness of people touched Jesus deeply. He did not have the callousness toward suffering we have developed as night after night we view suffering on television. Jesus cared.

In another reference we read that when Jesus saw a dumb and deaf man he sighed. An alternate translation is "he groaned." At the grave of Lazarus he sighed heavily. He was *deeply* moved. He cried.

Jesus suffers with us when we suffer. He groans. He sighs. He is deeply moved. He cries. Sometimes we actually can see him crying as one of his children sits at our bedside and cries because we are ill. Christ cries for us through that person, and thus his love becomes visible to us.

At the same time, Jesus the Healer is determined to heal. Over and over we read: "I will: be clean." "I will come and heal him." "Be healed."

So encompassing was Jesus' desire to heal that it appears at times to encircle masses of people. "Large crowds followed him, and he healed them there" (Matt. 19:2). He loved and loved. He could not do other than love, for he is love. He wished only well for people.

But though he ministered to the masses, Jesus never lost sight of the individual. Nor does Jesus the Healer ever lose sight of the individual patient in the hospital today, surrounded though one may be by hundreds of others. The patients may feel insignificant and lost. They know the medical staff identifies them mostly by the numbers on their wristbands. But the Healer doesn't need wristbands. The Healer asks permission to come into each room. He addresses each patient by name. He talks to each one individually, kindly, gently, and unhurriedly. He listens. He looks at the ill one closely. His hand smooths back the hair, holds the hand, tweaks the toe. The sick one who is full of fear he gathers into his arms and holds close, saying not a word but letting comfort and security pass from his body to the frightened one.

Jesus healed each of the ill ones differently. He told one to go to the priest, and in the going the man was healed. He told another to rise up, take up his bed, and walk. As the man struggled to his feet, he was healed. The Healer touched another. He put his fingers in the ears of one, and applied clay to another. As one sick person simply touched him, she was healed. To another he said simply, "My grace is sufficient for you," and enabled that follower to live with his infirmity. So too he deals with each one of us as he sees best.

The Healer healed, irrespective of race or status. Rich or poor, Roman, Jew, or Gentile—he reached out to all.

He disliked fanfare. He didn't want his healing ministry to become a public spectacle. Healing was simply one aspect of his service to people.

However, he accepted and even expected gratitude. Consider the story he told of the ten lepers. "Did only one come back to say thanks?" he asked. What tone do we hear in his voice as he speaks?

Jesus, the Healer, could heal because he had power to heal. He had received this power from the Father. "If I drive out demons by the finger of God, then the kingdom of God has come to you," he said (Luke 11:20).

Power also poured through him to others as he prayed. When Lazarus emerged from the grave, Jesus thanked his Father that his Father had heard his prayer (John 11:41).

When others drained him of power, Jesus turned to prayer for the restoration of power (Luke 6:12).

The Healer also recognized that sin was the primary evil that needed to be dealt with. He was not content with just healing people of physical ailments. He wanted people to know also that they could be set free from slavishly, selfishly serving their own interests and could become liberated, forgiven children of God.

"Which is easier," Jesus asked, "to say 'Your sins are forgiven,' or to say, 'Get up and walk'? But so that you may know that the Son of Man has authority on earth to forgive sins. . . ." Then he said to the paralytic, "Get up, take your mat and go home." And the man got up and went home (Matt. 9:5-7).

Certain Christian writers have helped us see this close connection between our being rightly related to God and being physically well. Vernon J. Bittner, E. Stanley Jones, and Norman Vincent Peale are among those who offer us much help. Peale, in his book *Dynamic Imaging,* writes: "I'm convinced that human beings are *supposed* to be healthy; we were *designed* to be healthy; that is what the Creator intended when he made us. I constantly image myself as a disease-free individual. It reminds me of something an airline pilot told me one day when he came back through the plane to visit with us passengers. I said to him, 'It always amazes me how these big planes stay up in the air. All this tremendous weight, all this fuel, all of these people, all their baggage. It is astonishing!'

" 'Not really,' the pilot said. 'It is the nature of airplanes to stay up in the air. They are designed to fly. They want to stay up in the air. It is very hard for a plane not to stay up in the air, because that is the way they are put together.'

"That is the way God put us together too. To be healthy,

energetic, creative, dynamic people at every age, full of vitality, and health. I'm sure of it. But we have a responsibility, too, not to abuse our bodies."

The early church recognized a close connection between living in a right relationship with God and health. When instructions were given for conducting healing services, confession of sin was acknowledged as an important prelude to healing.

"Is anyone of you sick? He should call the elders of the church to pray over him and anoint him with oil in the name of the Lord. And the prayer offered in faith will make the sick person well; the Lord will raise him up. If he has sinned, he will be forgiven. Therefore confess your sins to each other, and pray for each other so that you may be healed" (James 5:14-16).

This does not mean, however, that all illness is caused by a broken relationship with God. Job was deeply troubled because his friends were sure he was suffering because he had sinned. He acknowledged his sinfulness but insisted he was living in a right relationship with God. He admitted he couldn't understand either why he was suffering.

Perhaps in Job's case we can see his boils and sores as a natural consequence of all the stress he experienced through his multiple, sudden, traumatic losses. But the fact remains that Christians living in close relationship with God do get sick too. If we do not care for our bodies, we become more susceptible to illness, but caring for our health and walking in fellowship with God do not automatically guarantee us good health. God desires to heal, but at the same time God has given no promise that we shall not be ill—so ill that healing does not come, but death results instead. The New Testament tells us of saints who were ill or ailing and not healed.

Only when the kingdom of God comes finally and fully will we know freedom from sin, pain, disease, and death. The kingdom of God did come when Jesus came, ushering in a new era for the sick. But even as Jesus the King is coming, so too the kingdom is coming. It came. It is with us. And it will come. When it finally comes in its fullness, it will bring to an end all sickness.

So what do we do till then?

We look to Jesus, our Healer. He is by our side. He sees us. He stops. He sighs and groans and feels bad because we are sick. He asks us what we want him to do. He assures us he wants to help. And then he acts.

He deals with each of us differently. From one he removes a tumor, either surgically through the hands of a doctor or miraculously. He has power to do so. Another he recalls from apparent death. For another he heals broken bones. With yet another he deals tenderly, pointing out carefully coddled and nourished resentments and ill feelings that must be surrendered to him before healing can come. To another he gives the peace that relieves anxiety that, in turn, lessens pain. Another he enables to give up a destructive, competitive way of living, and the ulcers disappear. With yet another he groans as he sees disease twist limbs out of shape. He has the power to prevent it, but this time he does not use the power.

But however he chooses to deal with us, he is with us. We need not hesitate telling him what we would like him to do for us, trusting at the same time that he will give us the best. If we pray for healing once, and it is not granted, we need not hesitate to pray again the next time we become ill. Failure in other areas does not cause us to give up. Why then should seeming failure when we pray cause us to quit praying? We always can come to the Lord with any

141

concern. But as we come, we release our grip on what we are asking. We offer the Lord open hands, receptive hearts, and willing, submissive spirits. We do not bully or order God. We remember who we are and whom we are approaching.

If and when healing comes, we shall feel we are just beginning to understand the meaning of worship. Profound gratitude will spill over in love to God. We shall express that love by loving our bodies too, by nourishing them with wholesome food, by sending the blood racing through them as we exercise. We shall respect the limits of our bodies and allow them to relax and recuperate through rest. We shall care for our bodies, knowing that what we as individuals do for ourselves can be twice as effective as all the benefits of 20th-century medicine.

We shall treasure good mental health also and shall love our minds by stimulating them with new ideas. We shall seek to keep our dispositions sweet with humor and tolerance and by maintaining a forgiving spirit. We shall endeavor to keep growing by daring to take risks. We shall value our ability to be social creatures and cultivate new friendships and deepen old ties. We shall love work for its opportunities to express our true selves. We shall cherish our families and friends more than ever and place high priority on making strong the bonds that unite us. And because our hearts sing with joy in God our Savior we shall find ourselves loving even the unlovely and wanting to reach out to others. Conscious of the costly price that has been paid for our health and healing, we shall live ever aware of the fact that we have a debt to repay. We shall care for our health, but we shall not hoard it. Instead we shall use it in service.

And what if healing does not come to us? Even then we do not need to lose heart nor faith. We will believe that

God's grace *is* sufficient, that his power is made perfect in weakness. We shall look up, lift up our heads, and look for the coming of the King. With his coming will come also complete wholeness and vibrant health. And if he delays his coming, we shall look forward to being ushered into his presence through death. And then we shall be his people and God himself will be among us, and he will wipe away every tear from our eyes; and there will no longer be any death, there will no longer be any mourning, or crying, or pain, the first things will have passed away. Amen. Come, Lord Jesus.